Is there hope for ı
Is there a purpose

MW01199123

Tapping the eternal wisdom oj the ages, as well as her own stunning story and life-changing experience on the Other Side, Dr. Joyce reveals how you too can believe and receive miraculous results.

In this life-changing, paradigm-shifting book, Dr. Joyce Hunt Brown shares her extraordinary story of a life filled with unimaginable tragedy and miraculous triumph, horrendous heartache and heavenly happiness and joy. Now, at almost 90 years old, after conquering countless, overwhelming obstacles and crushing setbacks, Dr. Joyce has distilled the lessons of her long, miraculous life into one clear, compelling, desperately-needed message for today: You too can have a life filled with miracles. In *Amazing Heavenly Answers* you will:

1. Discover Your True Purpose for Living
2. Learn How to Unleash the Power of Your Miraculous Mind
3. Gain a Wondrous Cure for Depressed or Suicidal Thoughts
4. Learn Unique Techniques to Relieve Stress, Depression, & Grief
5. Explore Powerful Healing Practices for Your Mind and Body
6. Find Hope and Relief in the Midst of Your Most Challenging Circumstances
7. Learn to Draw on the Miraculous Powers of Heaven to Find Answers to Life's Most Pressing Problems

In this book, Dr. Joyce Brown also shares her astounding story of meeting God, the gifts she received from the experience, a divine message offering proof of God's unconditional love, the eternal wisdom that radically transformed, and gave new meaning and purpose to her life. As Dr. Joyce knows from her own experience, there is life after life. If you want to learn how to make sure you enjoy the Other Side when you get there, read this book.

Amazing Heavenly Answers[TM]
New Updated and Revised Edition

Earlier versions of this book include *God's Heavenly Answers* published in 2014 and *Heavenly Answers for Earthly Challenge* published in 1997. This edition has been extensively revised and updated.

10 9 8 7 6 5 4 3 2 1 0

Printed in the United States of America
ISBN 978-0-9913320-8-3 (Paperback)

Disclaimer: The content of this book is based on the author's own personal experiences and is for informational purposes only and is not intended to diagnose, treat, cure, or prevent any condition or disease, nor is it to replace the advice or care of professional health-care practitioners.

Hope Doctor Press
STRESS AND GRIEF RELIEF, INC.,
355 West Mesquite Blvd. Suite C-70, Mesquite, NV 89027
Phone: 1-800-734-3439 | Email: askwisdom@yahoo.com
www.StressAndGriefRelief.org & www.HopeDr.org

V031-PAPERBACK/HARDCOVER (Updated: June 23, 2023)

AMAZING HEAVENLY ANSWERS

How My Life After Life Experience Can Help You Find Hope, Love, and Peace

A True Story by
Dr. Joyce Hunt Brown, Ph.D., N.D., E.F.T.

Is there Hope for My Problems?

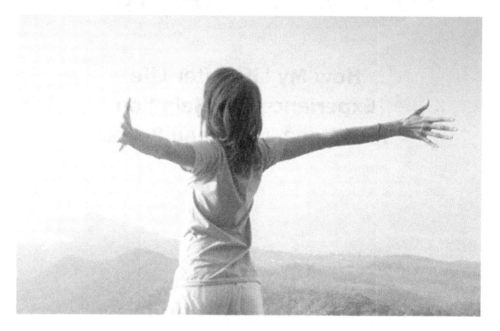

Is there a Purpose for Living?

What People Are Saying

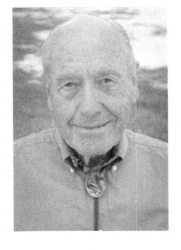

2016, I was termed an ALS reversal. Though I have not completely healed, we continue to enjoy life and move forward. This new book is valuable for anyone looking to improve their life in multiple ways and is totally inspiring. We hope you will read it."
—Kim and Kay Cherry,
Founders of ALS Winners

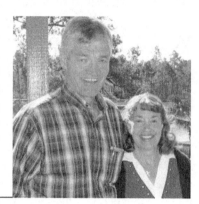

"I have firsthand knowledge that the book *Amazing Heavenly Answers* is actually saving lives. The author, Dr. Joyce Brown, shatters the myth that all you have to do is kill yourself to get a heavenly place of peace and beauty. Joyce's near-death experience of being on the Other Side convinced her that every day in this life is precious, that we can't win the prize if we take a shortcut and never finish the race, and that there is purpose to every life. Joyce was suicidal from the age of eight, and when her father committed suicide, she very nearly joined him. She often saw suicide as an option to escape the problems of this life, and consequently, often avoided the problem-solving process. Her experience on the Other Side changed her life forever. Her book should be read by every person who struggles with suicidal thoughts. To those in a position to make a difference, I hope you will lend your influence and help correct some of the false ideas that are rampant in our country. Joyce's files are steadily filling with letters from people whose lives have been saved by reading her book."

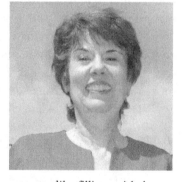

—Darla Isackson, *Finding Hope While Grieving Suicide*

"I have personally known Dr. Joyce Brown for many years and know her very well in all aspects of her life. I have known about her battles with pain, paralysis, Rheumatoid Arthritis, ALS, blindness, great financial losses, and the loss of loved ones. I know that it has helped her to learn patience, tolerance and the real value of health, relationships, and life. As she struggled with Agoraphobia, despair, stress, and betrayals, I believe this is why she is better able to feel compassion, empathy and a love for mankind. From my own personal experience, I know she understands better, firsthand, what so many others are going through. I have been a holistic health practitioner for over 30 years. I have learned from Joyce's near-death experience about God's special messages to prepare for my own Other Side's life review. Over all these years that I have known her, I have taken the opportunity to share with many people these eternal truths that she has taught. I have seen results people have had after Dr. Joyce conducted seminars, speaking engagements, coaching, and sharing her unique coping techniques, including anger management, and helping them overcome depression. She has guided people to take responsibilities for their lives and future, rather than blaming someone else for their problems and past mistakes, as they also found their own purpose for living. Dr. Joyce has had many productive counseling sessions with people of all ages, including working with the youth, and especially in detention centers and prisons in Utah and California where she shared her Other Side experience to sizable, captured, audiences. I'm still learning things from her many experiences and I consider her an eternal friend and believe we will know each other forever."

—**N. Louise Ferguson,** a close friend & colleague of Dr. Joyce

"The encouraging message in *Amazing Heavenly Answers* must be read by those who are struggling in the darkness of despair and sorrow. It is rich in wisdom and practical answers for all. This book is a self-contained support group!"

—**Kevin A. Brown,** Attorney at Law

"I want to thank Joyce Brown for putting things back in perspective for me. The day after I read this book (I read it in one sitting!), I viewed my life from a completely different, and much improved perspective. It's great to be reminded in such a compelling way about what really matters most—now and in eternity."

—**Janice Kapp Perry,** Author, Composer

"I've known Joyce Brown since before the events she describes in her book . . . I was aware of a marked change in her approach to life afterward.

She now handles difficulties and challenges with the confident attitude of one who has the peace of mind that comes from knowing her purpose and direction in life. Her story will greatly enrich the life of anyone who reads it."

—**S. Burt Chamberlain,** MSW, Ed.D.

"I have read everything I could find on near-death experiences for the last 32 years. This topic of what happens on the Other Side of our existence is very important, comforting, uplifting and interesting. It also gives knowledge of what's ahead of us. This book has all the answers to all the questions anyone will ever ask about what happens when one passes over to the Other Side of existence. Information contained in this book really gives answers to the reason why we are here and in this place. It tells us what consequences we face for our actions and what we should be thinking about and how we should live our lives every day. I recommend this as required reading for everyone!"

—**Devin Thomas**

"Thanks, Joyce, for writing this book. It is one of the most powerful and life-changing books I have ever read. It has given me a new understanding of life and how to enjoy the Other Side when I get there."

—**Jim Robbins** (Jim's quote after reading a previous edition just shortly before he passed. Jim is Tony Robbins' father.)

"About 5 years ago, I was blessed to meet Joyce Brown. She had given me her book (*Heavenly Answers*) to read. I was going through a lot at that time and I was addicted to drugs. I started reading the book, but ended up in jail before I could finish it. Joyce visited me in jail and arranged for me to receive another book so I could finish it, which I did while in custody. I can't tell you the power that book had in my life. I didn't get clean from drugs right away, but that book gave me hope and I no longer wanted to die. Now, I am 16 months clean and sober and am undergoing treatment for Hepatitis C. Some days are really rough and seem almost unbearable. But I make it through the day with the hope Joyce shares in her book. I believe in the message the book sends out to all those who are having a hard time in life. I encourage you to read her book. It had a life-changing effect on my life. I just want to say thank you, Joyce, for having the

courage to write this book. It has helped me immensely. I will always have a special place in my heart for you. Thank you."
—**Barbara Cimino,** Former drug addict

"Thank you for writing your book. It gave me a different perspective about life and my problems. Now I have found reasons why I want to live instead of automatically wishing I could die or wanting to trade places with someone else."
—**Michelle L,** Student, Age 14

Letters from Readers

When I wrote the first edition of this book and published it in 1997, I didn't know what to expect or how it would be received. But as letters came in from readers, I felt overwhelmed by their comments and the life-changing experiences they told me about. I lost many of the letters in the fire that ravaged my home, but I did recover a few and wanted to share some of their comments here in this new and updated version of my book in the hopes that others will find their comments helpful as well.

Dear Dr. Joyce,

Thank you so very much for coming into my life. You are an Angel sent from GOD. I thank you for your energies and your love. You are truly an inspiration to me, and it filters down to those I encounter. For such a blessing as you, I give thanks. You have helped so many people along the way. Dr. Joyce, I just want you to know that your book has been a BLESSING in my life, and for that I am truly grateful. Thank you, and may God forever bless you.

Sincerely,
—**Ruby deBraux**

Dear Joyce,

I have been suffering from severe bipolar and Post Traumatic Stress disorder for over 20 years. Countless times I have been lured by false hope that suicide would end my suffering. After several critical attempts and countless hospitalizations, I found your book. It was truly an answer to prayer!

Amazing Heavenly Answers contains life-saving facts for those contemplating suicide, and eternal truths that we ALL need in order to fully have the peace in the afterlife that we desire. I feel this book should be standard issue for everyone entering psychiatric treatment. If that were done, countless dollars, in-patient stays, and immeasurable human suffering could be eliminated. Also, this book is an invaluable tool for clergy of all faiths who so many times find themselves struggling to find effective counsel for those suffering in their congregations.

Your guidance regarding the urgency of proper use of time; the fact that we create our own heaven or hell, and the absolute necessity to take complete responsibility for our thoughts and actions are desperately needed messages in today's society. Truly, your book is a work of inspiration, capable of educating against many of the deadly misconceptions that haunt us, and giving our souls the necessary tools to reach for the greatest heights for which we were created.

Your book brings blessings to the reader on multiple levels. As I was reading about your life review, I found myself conducting a review of my own soul, and immediately identified shortcomings that I know could "bankrupt" me in the After Life. *Amazing Heavenly Answers* serves as a kind of After Life SAT exam: allowing us to find out if we have the "right stuff" to enter Heaven and have it be the nirvana we all want it to be.

Thank you so much for enduring the depths of darkness, and coming back to show us the path to that ultimate Light. I'm sure that because of this book, you will find your "Heavenly savings account" balance to be beyond your wildest dreams! I will be indebted to you forever.

Love in Truth,

—Betty M.

Dear Dr. Joyce,

I wanted to tell you about my friend who I used to work with. (I lost my job recently.) She has been struggling a lot through her life and relies on many depression and anxiety pills. I have been wanting her to read your book *Amazing Heavenly Answers* and I recently found the copy you gave me when you first wrote it. I knew it would help her in her life.

She lost her mom last year, a brother-in-law a couple of months ago, and her dog this week, who was like her child. She doesn't have any children and her dogs are her babies. She finally sat down to read your book this evening and she sent me a text telling me that she cannot express how much the book is touching her heart and speaking to her. She said it is exactly what she needed. She goes on to say that she is in awe and amazed and that it is the 3rd miracle she has experienced in her life. She said that God has answered her cries through the darkness by reading your book.

It has restored her faith and she is now crying tears of JOY. She says you are an amazing woman! Thank you for sharing your story. It is truly touching and does help those who are lost.

Love,

—Kari Peterson

Dear Joyce,

Thank you for writing your book. I read and re-read it often in order to convince myself that life is worth living, no matter how painful or difficult it gets. I have many extremely painful health problems. In fact, I have been to the Other Side myself. I had become too "heavenly minded to be any Earthly good" by wanting to be there instead of here.

After a series of tragedies causing me to lose almost everything, I didn't want to live anymore. Your book has helped me dramatically. It is such a strong and effective tool against suicide that I wrote letters and sent books to relatives, friends, and loved ones. I hope and pray your message will be spread by radio and TV interviews and even a movie.

Best wishes and thanks with all my heart,

—Sheila Wall

I cannot adequately put into words how profoundly your book *Amazing Heavenly Answers* touched my heart! I am inspired by your words. Thank you for sharing your insight and experience with the world. Your book really touched me at a time I needed to hear your message. Please, please, please keep marketing it—it is needed.

—Jan Snow, Marketing Manager,
PCS Multimedia Packaging

"Joyce is the most giving, loving and forgiving person I have ever known. Joyce's book *Amazing Heavenly Answers* confirms the movie, *The*

Greatest Story Ever Told, which was about Christ. I feel that her book stands along with the greatest books ever written because it is God's message."
—Ronald Runnells

Reviews of Amazing Heavenly Answers

Amazing Heavenly Answers conveys spiritual truths in a simple (but not simplistic) manner. Perhaps the outstanding feature of this book is not so much that it tells you entirely new revelations, but rather that which you feel inside that you have heard before, along with a spiritual sense of truth—a certain inspiration. Particularly recommended for those feeling depressed.

—Stacy Harlan

A couple of years ago I was given Dr. Joyce Brown's book *Amazing Heavenly Answers* by a patient of mine who strongly recommended to me that I had to read it. Within a week I had finished the book and was on the phone with Joyce discussing not only the book but her interest in the connection between oral health and disease and the rest of the human body. Joyce had been instructed, while she was out of her body, that the cause of her illness was a specific tooth that was diseased and the bacteria inhabiting the dead tooth were releasing toxins that were killing her. As we compared notes from her perspective as a patient, and mine as a doctor, we discovered that we were on common ground.

Since then, Joyce has been a good friend and ally in support of good oral health both in preventing dental disease and in treating it. We also share an interest in the soul of humanity, the physical connection to the spiritual that is the essence of her first book and has been the focus of her life since her return from death. This cannot be better stated than Tielhard de Chardin's words: "We are not human beings having a spiritual experience; we are spiritual beings having a human experience."

—Wendell Robertson, D.D.S., Biological Dentist

Dedication

This book is dedicated to all those who think life is not worth living. This is a book of hope, created to help each person find their own purpose for living.

Our mission is to change and save lives. Through our books, audiobooks, and other information products, we share proven, practical knowledge and timeless wisdom with people who need to overcome stress, grief, depression, health ailments, suicide, and more.

All proceeds from this book are donated to this cause.

Stress and Grief Relief, Inc., 501(c)(3) is a life changing, life saving non-profit organization. All donations are tax deductible (EIN: 95-472-2033).

Stress and Grief Relief, Inc.
355 West Mesquite Blvd. Suite C-70,
Mesquite, NV 89027.

1-800-734-3439
www.HopeDr.org

Table of Contents

Part Two

My Experience in the Spirit World

Part Three
My Life after I Returned to Earth

Appendices

Why I Wrote This Book: To Give You Hope—Death is Not the End, There is Life After Life

After pleading with God to die, and then getting a glimpse of Heaven and Hell, I knew I had to write this book. Death is not the end. There is life after life.

My life has been filled with challenges and calamities, but also many miracles. This is the story of my life before and after I died in 1983, and was given another chance to live with a new purpose. It is also about my life before and after being healed of ALS in 1988. Perhaps most importantly, this book is filled with the heavenly answers to earthly questions I have learned along the way, including the wisdom I've gained as a result of the many challenges I've conquered, and the stories around the many miracles I've received throughout my life.

In 1983, I returned to life as a transformed person, knowing I had a definite purpose for living and, therefore, that I had to make it through challenges rather than giving up because of them—and to help others do the same.

It is my hope that the answers I received and the wisdom I learned may be used by others in their own lives so they may find hope, healing and relief from stress, depression and grief. Having lost my father, sister, and other family members to suicide, as well as the death of other family and friends, I understand the grief that comes from losing loved ones and others you sincerely care about.

One of the most encouraging things I found when I was on the Other Side is that we *will* see our loved ones again. If we could just hear the message they are trying to tell us, we would know how much they care, and how much they want us to use our remaining time wisely.

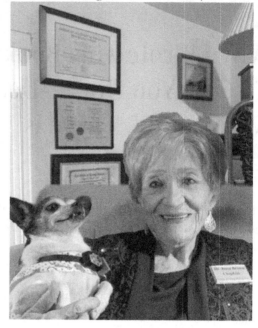

Since COVID-19 has raged around the world, there has been a huge increase in depression, anxiety, and grief, both from the loss of friends and loved ones, but also from the extreme changes the virus has forced us to endure. All of this has led to an unprecedented rise in suicides.

Regardless of the problems we are facing, there are no easy solutions. The answers are the same as those I found for the multiple problems, challenges and calamities I faced during my life. The only way we can improve our situations is by getting control of our thoughts, feelings, and actions, with courage, faith, hope, and a *definite chief purpose for living*. We need to endure as best we can, one hour at a time if need be. As we seek relief from stress and grief, call upon the powers of Heaven, and help and serve others, we may reap miracles.

This book is written from my heart to yours.

Truly, with Divine intervention, I have cheated death numerous times, including surviving car accidents, overcoming major illnesses, living through other life-threatening disastrous events, as well as actually dying and returning to my body.

Since 1981, millions of near-death experiences (NDE) have been reported. Psychiatry researchers Linda J. Griffith and Bruce Greyson estimate that five percent of the adult American population has reported having a near-death experience. The Near-Death Experience Research

Foundation (NDERF) reports that nearly 800 NDEs occur every day in the U.S. As a result of people coming forward, these profound, transformational life experiences are becoming more well-known to the general public.

In his book, *The Republic*, the ancient Greek philosopher Plato recounts the first known description of a Near Death Experience. In a section at the end of Book X known as "The Myth of Er," Plato tells of an incident involving a soldier named Er who was killed in battle and believed to be dead. Ten days later when Er and the other bodies of the dead were about to be taken up, Er's body was found without corruption or decay. When Er was about to be buried, he revived and told the onlookers of his experience in the Other World. Er tells of the great consequences, but also great rewards given to the souls he saw, each according to how they had lived their lives.

It's surprising how many people I have personally met after sharing my story of dying and going to the Other Side who told me they too had a near-death experience. There are commonalties, yet each experience is unique and different in their own ways.

Scores of books have been written about people's experiences, including several by Arvin Gibson and David Bennett. Arvin Gibson was a good friend and mentor. He greatly encouraged me to get my book, *Heavenly Answers*, written and published. Afterward, he told me he felt that my book contained special NDE information that people would want to know and read about for years after we are both gone.

He was also instrumental in helping the world become more aware of the many near-death experiences that were being reported. Although Arvin didn't have a near-death experience himself, he was fascinated by the phenomenon. Before he wrote each of his books, he would interview dozens of people who had a near-death experience. He would choose the most interesting stories, and then verify their information before including them in his books.

He found during their experience they had many things in common, which he then documented. Some describe going through a tunnel, others are just up and out of their bodies as I was. They all realized they were in a different realm. Most meet a bright, white light and they have an overwhelming knowledge that God is real. Earth life is not the true world.

Most people who have an NDE have a panoramic life review, which gives them a new perspective of their own life on Earth, and reasons to make it through challenges.

Some wanted to stay on the Other Side, but were told they had to go back. They had not finished their purpose for living, which could affect generations to come. Others wanted to return to Earth life because they felt they were needed by family and friends.

One of the telltale signs of someone having a near-death experience is when they come back a transformed person, with a driving purpose for living and a desire to share it with all who will listen.

When interviewing people, Arvin discovered almost all of the near-death survivors had the same belief as to who God is, just as they did before they had their NDE.

The case of Howard Storm is an interesting exception. Storm wrote a book about his experience titled: *My Descent into Death*. He died a confirmed atheist. He descended into what he described as Hell after his death. He then called upon Jesus Christ to save him. He came back to life a confirmed Christian and became pastor of a church.

The International Association for Near-Death Studies (IANDS) has group leaders and chapters all over the world where people can go and tell about their unique NDE, and where those interested can go to listen. I've been an IANDS group leader for several years.

David Bennett, the IANDS Groups Coordinator and Board Member at Large also had a fascinating, in-depth near-death experience. With the knowledge and determination he gained from having been on the Other Side, he was able to completely heal himself within six months of the time he was diagnosed with stage IV lung cancer. David has written several books, including *Voyage of Purpose*, and remains very active with the IANDS organization.

Having a near-death experience is a great life changing miracle. We all have many more miracles than we realize. Not until we are on the Other Side, and are able to see each of our own lives from an eternal perspective, will we be able to know just how many miracles we have each had.

I have had many miracles and you can too. As I share some of my miraculous experiences, perhaps it will inspire you with additional hope and faith to receive miracles as well. I know of countless others who have received miracles, a number of which you will learn more about toward the end of this book (see Conquering Heroes section), and, through my non-profit work, I continue to meet new people and hear new stories of still others who have received miracles.

Usually, in order to receive miracles, we have to do all that we can. This includes a number of things I have learned and will share with you in this book, including unique coping techniques for life's various challenges, as well as for stress, grief relief, depression, and even suicide prevention. Miracles, I have found, are preceded by a number of things, including positive beliefs and actions, but even more importantly, having courage, faith and really trusting in and listening to God. Utilizing this information can also help you gain eternal peace of mind.

Part One

My Life
Before Being on the
Other Side

CHAPTER 2

Rock Fights and Bullies

This is where my story begins.

From the time I was a small child, I felt unloved, unwanted and that I was a big burden for having been born. I was born in the fall of 1933 during the Great Depression. My father did not want me because I was not a boy.

When I was about eighteen months old, he dropped my mother and me off at her parents' farm. He left us there with no means of support, and he never came back.

My parents divorced soon after. I remember seeing my father perhaps three or four times during my childhood.

As soon as she was able, my mother moved us to Pocatello, Idaho. It was still during the Great Depression. Many banks and businesses were closed, jobs were scarce, and millions struggled just to get food. Mother found a job scrubbing floors at a hotel.

She told me that there were many times she had to leave me crying in a bathtub, but she had no choice. She was so busy as a struggling single mom, trying to make a living and take care of us.

She was often sad, and cried a lot. When I was three or four years old, I remember sitting in a little rocking chair just wanting to be good and not cause problems that would make Mother feel worse.

In addition, I had bad cases of whooping cough, mumps and measles, and the whole time feared I might make my mother cry. Chicken pox at least waited until I was much older.

Being an only child, without other family for guidance or direction, I felt confused, lonely and unhappy. At times, I just wanted to disappear. But, I didn't realize how hard this situation was on my mother, too.

When I was not quite six years old, I started school in first grade. I knew I didn't fit in. The other kids didn't like me. They made fun of my clothes. When I walked, they could see my shoes had cardboard in them to cover the holes in the bottoms. After only about two weeks of school, I told the teacher I was quitting and not coming back any more. I told her I had learned to sign my name, count my money, and I didn't need to learn anything else.

I did not know where I was going to get the money I would be counting, but I thoroughly believed that was all I needed to know.

The next thing I knew, they had contacted my mother to come in and talk to the principal. I remember sitting on a bench outside the office while they were talking. I felt this was a useless meeting. I had made up my mind. I was not going to school any more. When they came out of their meeting, they informed me I was going back to school for many years to come. When I heard their decision, it made me cry. Unhappily, I realized they could force me to go to school, but my mind and heart would not be there.

It was many years of wasted time in my life before I discovered the value of learning and education. With my mother so busy having to work and with her own problems, I felt like an orphan and a big burden to her throughout my life.

When I was six and a half years old, a family friend seriously molested me. This just added to my confusion and unhappiness. My mother did not believe me, which created more hurt. With all the difficulties she was going through, I don't think she realized how serious it was.

When I was in second grade, 7 years old, one day at school, the teacher came down to my desk and asked me a question about our lesson that day. I had not fully understood the question. When I didn't give the answer she wanted, she got angry and suddenly struck me with her cupped hand on the left side of my head, right over my ear. Immediately, I heard a loud ringing and lost a large part of my hearing. This caused permanent damage. The situation was basically ignored.

However, by the sixth grade, the principal and teachers decided I needed to take lip-reading classes which I did for the next four years. They greatly helped compensate for my hearing loss.

When I was eight years old, my mother took me with her to a funeral. They talked about how happy the person was who died and how nice it is in Heaven. They spoke as if they KNEW this for certain, as if they had all been there before.

8

It sounded wonderful. About a month later, I learned about suicide and decided that it was what I wanted to do, believing I could just go and be happy in Heaven. I am a very practical person. Why stay in this world with all of its problems, if I could just die and go to Heaven and be happy?

From this point on, giving up and thinking of going to Heaven became a way of life.

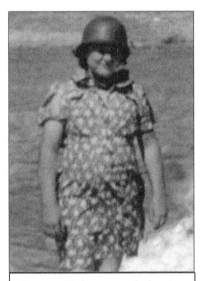

Joyce with her army helmet as protection from bullies with rocks.

When I was about ten years old some information surfaced and Mother told me she now believed I had been molested. I knew she was deeply sorry about it. She hadn't realized how bad it was and how much it affected me, but with all that was going on in her life at the time, she did not know what to do about it. I was glad she at least acknowledged it.

However, I had mentally moved on and by this time I had new problems. As an overweight and combative child, I was bullied and was the brunt of schoolyard jokes.

My weight and lack of nice clothes led to a great deal of painful teasing, taunting, and rejection. I was the brunt of almost everyone's humor. Having a lot of energy, I often used it in unproductive directions that brought me many hurtful experiences. It seemed I was always in a fight of some sort. Being a natural fighter both helped and hurt me. I even wore an army helmet that protected my head during rock fights with the neighbor kids. I didn't start them, but after they began, I hung in there until they ended.

Gradually, however, I lost a lot of my enthusiasm and kept to myself most of the time. One morning, also at age ten, I woke up with severe pain in my side and was sick to my stomach. Mother took me to the doctor, who admitted me to the hospital. They had no time to tell me what was happening, and I was naturally afraid.

As I was on a gurney being wheeled down to the operating room, a nurse looked down at me and said in a loud voice, "She is so fat. She's

9

huge." For a 10-year old not knowing what was happening, that was devastating.

Tears began to roll down my face, and by the time we got to the operating room, I was sobbing with fright and embarrassment.

People need to realize that words can hit as hard as a fist. I found out after my surgery that my appendix was about to burst. This was one of my first of many miracles.

CHAPTER 3

Troubled Teens and More Miracles

At age 12, I had a case of rheumatic fever that was so severe it was a miracle I survived. For a few years afterwards, it left me with weaknesses and complications. I was no longer able to ride a bike, climb stairs, or take physical education in school. However, miraculously, during my teen years, I recovered my strength, and did not have any long-term complications.

As I grew into a young woman, I became shy, anxious, fearful, and reclusive. When I was about 15, I came down with a severe case of chicken pox that lasted over three weeks, which added to my feelings of loneliness and depression.

I did not understand why God would not let me die. I had prayed and prayed that He would please take me to Heaven. Suicide was always in the back of my mind.

Within a few months, I turned 16 and my mother had remarried. I felt even more out of place. I called and made arrangements to go live with my father in Idaho, even though I hadn't seen him in years. He had remarried and I had a half-brother and a half-sister who were about 4 and 5 years old.

Things went well for the first few days. I enjoyed visiting with some cousins I hadn't met before. I thought this was a dream come true. It felt like I finally was part of a family.

One day while visiting with a cousin, we had a big argument. I don't remember what it was about, but seemed very important at the time. I went back to the house where I was living with my dad, the family had just sat down to eat dinner.

When I came in, I told my dad about the argument with my cousin. He jumped up, grabbed hold of my clothes, threw me over into a corner of the room, and made me stand with my face to the wall. He said, I should have been able to solve all my own problems. I was not to come home a loser.

I stood in the corner, went without dinner and felt devastated, crushed and embarrassed, sobbing as they started eating. Dreams of having a life

11

with my father had just crashed down around me. After the meal was over, I was permitted to go to bed with no dinner.

The next day, my dad told me he had a car he needed me to drive. He explained that it wasn't registered and, to avoid being ticketed, he wanted me to follow him through the back roads, which meant going up a mountain on a single lane dirt road.

Even though I was frightened, and didn't want to drive the car, I didn't dare tell him no. It was winter and the roads were icy. Also, I had just barely gotten my driver's license, and had never driven on ice or snow.

As I followed him on back roads, we finally came to a rather steep mountain road. Almost at the top of the hill, the car began to slide backwards on the ice. Within seconds, the car was careening toward the edge of the road. Inches from the edge, with no guardrail, was a two or three hundred foot drop off. I could barely see the bottom over the side.

No matter what I tried to do, no matter how much or how little I pressed the gas pedal, the car just continued to slide toward the edge. The brakes wouldn't hold either. The car just kept sliding. I gripped the steering wheel tightly, closing my eyes and waiting for the fall to come.

Suddenly, out of nowhere, I felt a big bang on the back of the car. I looked in the rearview mirror, and saw a huge Idaho Power truck. It seemed to come out of nowhere. The driver began pushing my car back up on the road and over the top of the hill. I couldn't believe it! I was saved!

Once I knew for sure that I was safe and free of the ice, I was going to pull over to thank the driver for saving my life. But when I looked up into the rearview mirror, the truck was gone. It just vanished. I kept thinking how there were no side streets, and how it was impossible that he could have turned around on such a narrow road.

I soon decided it must have been a life-saving gift from God. I didn't realize it at the time, but this was one of my life's many miracles. Apparently, I had not yet fulfilled my life's purpose.

Within the next few days, I begged my mother, who finally agreed to let me come back home to live with her.

During my teen years I did lose weight, to the point that I developed an eating disorder, and became anorexic.

CHAPTER 4

Father's Near-Death Experience

At age 17, my father was traveling through a city nearby and was in a serious car accident. I went to visit him in the hospital.

He told me that during the accident he left his body and looked down, watching as the medics were working on him.

He also told me beauty and peace surrounded him, and he did not want to come back to life. This only reinforced my belief about Heaven, and my wish to die and go there.

At that time, I did not know that this beauty and peace he described is for people who have earned it during their limited Earth life, and who die in God's timing, not their own.

CHAPTER 5

From the Frying Pan to the Fire

For my 18th birthday, using money I had earned from helping a neighbor clean her house, I went to a diner, sat on a stool at the counter, and ordered cake and ice cream to celebrate. While I was sitting there, a handsome cab driver sat next to me. He ordered coffee and lit his cigarette.

A few puffs later, he started up a conversation. His words were very charming, and he had big blue eyes like my father's. I soon agreed to a date even though he was 11 years older than I was. After the date and more charming words, I fell head over heels in love.

When he proposed, this seemed like the perfect way to escape my unhappy home life. Two and a half weeks after our first meeting, we were married. However, right away I realized that my Prince Charming and I had nothing in common and were sorrowfully incompatible.

In addition, I now had a 7-year-old stepson from my husband's previous marriage. He was a sweet little boy, but, having just turned eighteen, I didn't have much experience even being around small children. I had no idea how to be a mother, let alone a step-mother—especially with all the other challenges we had in our marriage.

I had just jumped out of the frying pan, and into the fire.

Moving back home with my mother was not an option. I had to figure out how I could get out of this regrettable marriage. I felt desperately trapped.

Not knowing what else to do, I frantically called the clergy and asked him if there was any way he could not file that marriage certificate. I did not realize the legal entanglements to get out of an ill-fated marriage.

One of the very most important decisions a person can make is choosing a proper mate to spend their life with. What will their family life be like together? Will it be loving and fulfilling or filled with regrets, heartaches, and abuse?

CHAPTER 6

If Only...

By the time I was eighteen, my weight was normal and I had married, but not happily. My feelings of shyness intensified as I became more withdrawn than ever and shied away from people. My favorite outfit—a black scarf, a long maroon coat, and knee-high black galoshes with big zippers down the sides—made me feel invisible to the world.

Fear, dread of living, and feeling frightened of people were my constant companions, even when I wanted to go out to get the mail or the paper. I would peek out the drapes to see if anyone was around, then run out, get the paper or mail, and dash back into the house. My self-conscious and anxious feelings about meeting people or being seen by them were that intense—I was terrified of people!

On my nineteenth birthday I remember feeling exceptionally depressed. I felt "stuck," and I didn't see how my life could ever get any better. At 19, I was pregnant. In addition to caring for my step-son, to earn money for the family, I tended an

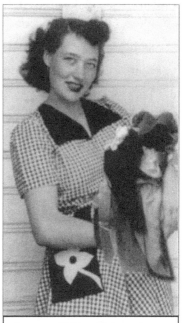

Joyce with family laundry at age 19.

additional three children day and night, whose mothers had health problems. Their ages were about four to eight years old. On top of all this I had the many challenges of being pregnant, including morning-sickness.

I took care of them 24 hours a day for several months. Unfortunately, all four children came down with chicken pox at about the same time. At least there was the miracle that I had already had chicken pox.

I hated life and I continually prayed to God that I would die. At 19 years old, I felt my life was hopeless.

As if this were not enough stress, my husband's brother and one of his friends also moved in with us.

I was cooking, baking homemade bread, and cleaning for all of us on top of being pregnant.

I vividly remember feeling extremely overwhelmed and depressed. There was no way for me to get out of this situation. I was trapped. Repeatedly, I pleaded with God to let me die. I harbored the false belief that my death was the only answer to all my problems.

My thoughts were full of "if only."

If only I had not gotten married so young without really knowing the man with whom I was to spend my life.

If only I had chosen a compatible husband with mutual interests and goals.

If only I had a better education so I could support my expected new baby and myself.

If only I could disappear and DIE.

I prayed and prayed to God to become a new person. If I was not going to die, please just help me to change.

Now as I share my experience with the youth, I plead with them to learn from my mistakes.

CHAPTER 7

A Life Changing Miracle

Finally, after several years, thinking over my miserable life to this point, and wanting to become a completely different person, a new miracle came into my life.

Praying and praying, I soon discovered unique *sleep learning* courses that, as I listened to them, changed my negative thinking to positive feelings and actions.

I desperately, and with *consistent* determination, listened to them day and night.

I gained new confidence and direction as the constant repetitions of positive affirmations reprogrammed my negative thinking.

It worked dramatic wonders in my life, and I had new confidence and self-esteem. For a brief time, I even did some modeling on TV, and in the newspaper.

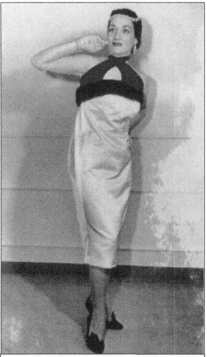

Joyce modeling after her changes from sleep learning.

After I learned I was expected to attend a party as an escort to one of the executives, I turned down a lucrative contract for a cigarette company. After one too many of these sort of requests, I soon realized there was no future for me in modeling.

CHAPTER 8

Life as a Single Mom

Unfortunately, I had married young, like my mother, and was terrified of becoming a single mom as she had been.

After about eight years in this heartbreaking marriage, I had three wonderful children, two daughters and a son. However, the situation was too overwhelming. Finally, in the fall of 1959, at the age of 26, I managed to get a divorce.

I found out the hard way, by not choosing to marry the right, compatible companion, usually separation and a bitter divorce will follow. Divorce can cause a loss of happy, family times together, disrupted and lonely holiday seasons, and the loss of close family ties from then on. This loss of family closeness may even include being almost totally alone for end-of-life care.

Most divorces can leave traumatic effects on the family.

CHAPTER 9

The Power of Sleep Learning: How Can We Learn While We Sleep?

Every night when we go to sleep, our conscious mind goes to sleep. Our subconscious mind, however, is awake and able to accept positive affirmations. This changes our thoughts and feelings, and helps create our ideal self, with potential for miraculous results. It did this for me, and countless others. It can do it for you, too.

By using an effective *sleep learning* system, with powerful positive affirmations, you can unconsciously change your self-talk which can change your life, helping you become your ideal self.

How often have you heard the expression, "Let me sleep on it"? Whether people realize it or not, our unconscious minds are continuously working to help us make decisions

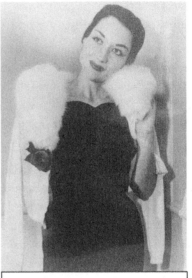

Joyce modeling on television.

and solve problems, even while we sleep. What most people do not realize is that you can work more effectively with your unconscious mind to better tap your brain's miraculous power.

In fact, with *sleep learning,* you can implant into your unconscious mind proper suggestions and thought patterns of courage, confidence, and right thinking, feelings, and actions which later benefit your everyday, conscious living. *Desire, visualize* and, with the help of God, you can *realize* miraculous results in your life.

As I continued to listen to the *sleep learning* courses, I began to replace my negative thinking with positive beliefs while I slept or meditated. They helped me to move forward with new confidence and determination.

I became a new, vibrant person. My memory increased to where I had an almost photographic memory. A test confirmed my ability to speed read at over 950 words per minute with near perfect comprehension.

Hard Work with Winning Results

To earn income, I decided I would become a real estate agent when I saw the high demand for newly-built homes. I studied real estate for a short time, and I passed the exam easily. I became a licensed real estate agent. The future looked promising.

I then determined which company had the highest sales and made an appointment to apply. The sales manager who interviewed me was adamantly against women in sales with his company. For over three hours we had a "friendly debate" as he gave excuses why women would not do well selling houses not yet built, and I responded with reasons why women could do at least as well, or even better than men. Finally, he decided to let me try.

Two of the five other sales*men* in the office openly joked to each other about me working there, saying how foolish it was for me or any other woman to even attempt to compete with them. We all participated in a contest of the month with our names and the number of sales we made on a large blackboard in the office.

I spent every free moment I could in the model home and calling on prospective leads. My hard work paid off when I won the contest for several months in a row. (Finally, the contest was terminated.) The two salesmen who had taunted me when I was hired, quit. I was surprised and pleased when I was introduced to the women who were their replacements.

I was beginning to understand the remarkable power of the human mind. It really is astonishing what you can do *when your mind is working for you instead of against you.*

My financial situation had improved considerably, but I was not able to keep up with the constant physical demands of selling real estate and was forced to resign. Not sure what direction my life would take, I continued my education by taking university classes when I could. Yet thinking about my future was still a big concern. More years of personal challenges went by as I kept studying and looking for ways to succeed in life.

CHAPTER 10

Tragic Auto Accident and After-Effects

In July of 1960, at the age of 27, because of a careless driver, I was seriously injured in a terrible car accident. Even though I had a lot of severe pain from the whiplash, and a serious injury to my lower back, I had to endure it for a year and a half before the driver's insurance would pay for the cervical neck and lower back surgery. By not having a very good attorney, I was disappointed that the money barely covered the attorney's costs, the doctors and the hospital. Also, I had lost precious time with my children while I recovered.

During such complicated surgeries and recoveries my children had to be cared for by others. I simply was not physically able to care for them myself.

When they operated, they found there were two herniated disks which required bone fusions. They surgically obtained the donor bone from my hip to fuse into my neck. Recovery from the hip surgery was more painful and complicated and greatly delayed my recovery and made it difficult to even get in and out of bed.

About two months later, I thought I was making great progress after the surgery. I drove to the store for some essential items. While I was stopped for a red light, the unimaginable happened. Unexpectedly, a car crashed into the back of mine. My neck snapped backwards causing another whiplash and broke loose the two previous fusions.

This ultimately required another two cervical neck fusions, and another donor bone surgery from my other hip. This involved additional recovery time and prolonged incapacitation. From my previous experience, and to avoid disheartening attorneys, court involvement and delays, I accepted their discouragingly low offer of only $6,000 and arranged for the payments to go directly to the doctors and hospital.

This additional surgery resulted in more time delays, and required a longer recovery with both hips painfully disabled.

I had to have eight major spinal surgeries over the next fifteen years that ended up being very traumatic and unsuccessful. Four of them were bone fusions in the neck and cervical area, and four were in the lower spine.

As a result, I was almost constantly in tremendous pain. My circumstances during this time were indescribably difficult to bear, including extreme spinal and balance problems that continue to this day.

After the tragic auto accident, and between surgeries, there were family situations in which I was overwhelmed as a single mom in this fragile condition caring for my children. I was very depressed, worried about their future, and missed my children terribly while going through this nightmare situation. My heart ached not being able to be with them.

Recently, when I was going through some old files, I found a poem I wrote expressing how I felt at the time:

My Prayer

Oh, my Father in Heaven above.
　　Show me Thy mercy and Thy love.
Things have happened here in my life.
　　Which have caused me much grief and strife.

My strength is gone. My spirit is weak.
　　And of your power and help I seek.
My mortal eyes just cannot see,
　　Any way that is left open to me.

To solve these problems that are so great
　　That will control my future and my fate
Must I be so terribly distraught,
　　Without thy guidance my hope is naught.

Three little spirits you've given to me
　　To guide and direct till they return to Thee.
Their cries ring loudly in my ears,
　　But I'm too far away to soothe their fears.

Oh God, be with them and comfort their souls

That the spirits of evil won't take their tolls.
Help us to conquer this illness and pain
        The cause of the separation of which I disdain.

Help us to meet these greatly mounting debts
        Which have added so much to our sorrows and frets.
How I ache for my three babies so fair.
        To hold them close so they know I still care.

Father bless us with health and strength,
        That we may enjoy life to a good length.
Grant us the ability, determination and drive
        To live more Christ-like as long as we're alive.

God, I'd humbly ask and I pray,
        If it can be Thy will, that maybe today
An answer might come.

Joyce Hunt (1962)

CHAPTER 11

Keep On Keeping On

There were some good times where it seemed my life was going to be much better. I thought about the story I'd heard of two frogs in a bucket of cream. They could not get out. One of them gave up, fell to the bottom, and drowned. The other was determined to keep swimming. As he paddled and paddled, he turned the cream to butter, and was able to jump out.

But then there were sudden, unexpected down turns between surgeries where it seemed impossible for me to endure. Tragic life events crashed down on me, compounding my sorrows and heartaches, reinforcing my belief that suicide was the only answer.

I felt trapped and needed to gain control of my thinking no matter the pain or how many problems I had.

Fortunately, throughout this period, I continued listening to the *sleep learning* recordings to create miracles and to get out of this situation and live a better life. Every time I went to the hospital for surgery, I took my special record player and *sleep learning* recordings, which helped with relaxation, pain relief and to prevent depression because of my situation. It was so important for me to keep up with the positive thinking and hope for a better future. I wanted to receive mental miracles.

I always felt more relaxed and less stressed as I listened to positive affirmations, such as: "I am calm, I am serene, I am confident, I enjoy life. I feel health and well-being all through my mind and my body."

Unfortunately, even with all the positive thinking, *sleep learning* didn't change my belief in the myth that all I had to do was die in order to receive an unearned peace.

Frustration, despair, and despondency took over because of the pain of so many surgeries. All of this led me to feelings of hopelessness, deep depression, and two failed suicide attempts. I just wanted to die.

At that time, I did not know that sometimes we can get so wrapped up in the present that we do not realize the future can hold wondrous changes.

There were other difficult and challenging situations, but I had progressed to where I no longer blamed God for unwanted circumstances. I had begun to realize that most of my problems were linked to my choices or my family's choices and without God's blessings things could have been much worse.

Botched Spinal Surgery

In the spring of 1973 at age 39, a lumbar, lower back surgery by a surgeon I will refer to as "Dr. B," dramatically changed my life forever. This horrifically botched surgery caused continuous excruciating pain and dropped foot.

After I was released from the hospital, I was required to wear a leg and foot brace in order to walk at all. This surgery was so outlandish and bizarre that it was suspected the surgeon was using illegal drugs.

Sometimes the more things seem hopeless, the bigger the miracle is needed, but we just have to "keep on keeping on."

Another Development

For several years prior to this, I had been consulting my gynecologist regarding additional health difficulties. He told me he believed my symptoms could have been cancerous.

I finally agreed to set aside some time in January 1974 to go to the hospital for exploratory surgery. He did find giant cysts that needed to be surgically removed, but none were cancerous. Even though it was good news, it required additional weeks of limited activity while I was recovering.

CHAPTER 12

After Effects of the Botched Spinal Surgery

Toward the first of June, 1974, at the age of 40, after desperately searching, I finally found an orthopedic surgeon who agreed to try to help reverse the extensive injuries caused by "Dr. B."

The damage to my spinal cord and the paralysis was so serious he did not know if he could help me.

The surgery took several hours and was partially successful for relieving some of the pain and paralysis. However, it was such a small amount that I could hardly tell the difference.

Right after the surgery, while I was still waking from the anesthetic in the recovery room, the surgeon came in to see me. Somehow, I knew, and I told him emphatically, that he had not gotten all of the sutures off which were wrapped around my spinal cord.

He answered me, "You can't know that. And we did get them all."

After about a year of extreme pain, and pleading with the Doctors to do a special test, that would determine whether there was still pressure on the spinal cord, they finally agreed, just to pacify me, and did it.

They were shocked to find out that what I was saying was true. It showed on the fluoroscope and the X-rays they had not gotten all the sutures off and there was still significant pressure on my spinal cord.

After the tests, one of the doctors came in the room and told me that for legal reasons they would all have to resign, and could not talk to me about my case any further. It would be up to me to find a different orthopedic surgeon for additional treatments for my spinal condition.

Prayers for Life or Death

For the next several months, I was still left with extreme pain and lost most of the use of my left leg and foot. I felt dismay, despair, and wondered what I could do.

Being a very active person, this greatly slowed me down, but did not stop me. A short time later, continuing to search for another surgeon, I went to the neurology department at a top university with my x-rays. Along the way, I stopped at a photography shop and had black and white copies made of the x-rays, which I still have today.

After their neurology team examined me and studied the x-rays, their top neurologist said words no one ever wants to hear. Tears welled up, and my heart almost stopped as I heard them say, "Your condition is hopeless and nothing more can be done." I simply needed to accept the fact that I was disabled and would just have to live with the paralysis and pain for the rest of my life.

Driving home, I was baffled and devastated. I could not believe what I had just been told. Arriving home, my mother was anxious to hear what the doctors had to say. She was expecting good news, that they could help me. She and I both cried, wondering what the future would hold. What in the world was I going to do?

I could not accept the doctors' pronouncement, or their finality of my condition and future. At that time, I felt I had to find a better answer or die. My prayers for relief or death seemed to go unheard and unanswered.

Positive Belief

My situation seemed futile. However, I continued searching for another surgeon for a year and a half.

Fortunately, there was nothing wrong with my right foot and leg and I was very capable of driving.

Finally, in late fall of 1975, at age 42, I found a top rated, highly recommended orthopedic surgeon. He agreed the surgery was needed in an effort to relieve some of the remaining damage and pressure on my spinal cord.

The extensive surgery was performed, including a massive donated bone graft fusion.

A week after this surgery, I went home. My leg and foot seemed much better. However, complications developed with my lower back area. I did not think my back pain could get any worse. But within a short time, a more painful condition of undetermined origin set in.

Unable to tolerate this new, worsening spinal condition, I called the doctor who made arrangements with the ambulance to pick me up and readmit me to the hospital.

The anticipation of being moved was almost intolerable, but as the medical technicians took me down the steps on the gurney, the unthinkable happened.

They dropped me. I nearly passed out.

After being admitted to the hospital, additional specialists were called in.

Soon, the most sophisticated tests that were available at the time were performed, but it was all to no avail.

It seemed that I would be permanently left in this agonizing state of existence with only the use of my arms, hands, mind, and voice.

The muscles in my body were atrophying at an accelerating speed. My leg muscles hung shriveled and limp from my protruding bones from not being able to move.

My doctor, a renowned orthopedic surgeon, a marvelous man whom I greatly appreciated and respected, delivered this heartrending message to me himself. The hospital's policy was that a patient could not remain in their care under hopeless conditions. I was told that my hospital room had to be vacated for someone with hope of recovery.

He had already made arrangements with a nursing home without telling me. A gurney was brought to take me by ambulance to my new residence.

Even though I was feeling shock and dismay, I asked my doctor if he believed in God.

When he replied that he did, I said, "I need more time; I will walk again. I believe in miracles."

I was still continuously listening to my *sleep learning* recordings to help reinforce my willed determination for my body to heal and walk again. I knew that with courage, faith, prayer, and positive thinking I would receive miracles.

It's amazing, the miraculous results that can be achieved by having faith, praying, and searching for answers rather than giving up. I did not accept what I was told about my condition.

Knowing how much my mom, and my now four-year old granddaughter, Crystal, needed me, I thoroughly believed I would recover and would even walk again. My mom and Crystal were a tremendous help during my surgery recovery and my heart is filled with gratitude and appreciation for both.

When my mental attitude was down and depressed, I wanted to die; when it was up, as it was then, I believed in miracles. I didn't realize how much my moods and thoughts affected other family members and those around me.

CHAPTER 13

Seeking Solutions and Making Progress

Having been granted additional time for recovery in the hospital, I didn't like just lying in bed being bored. I heard a nurse talking about a fun gift available on the east coast, a little plastic object being sold as a new type of "sea pet."

My mind was sparked with ideas. I thought of a pebble being a perfect, constant-companion pet. Most pets take a lot of care; this one would not. It was getting close to the holidays, and since I could not get out to shop, I thought this would make a good Christmas gift for some of my family and friends.

In spite of my pain, I felt exuberant as I thought of ideas about what to call these new pets and how to care for them. Not wanting to portray them as just plain old rock-pebbles, I wrote of them as unique pets. Suddenly I thought of their name, *Pedigreed Pet Pebbles.*™

They Bring Good Luck

Ideas continued coming to my mind. Grabbing a pen and paper, I began to write. The words flowed quickly: "Genuine, unique Pedigreed Pebbles™—the Perfect Pets." I described how they could bring good luck, how loyal they were, and that they had a long life expectancy.

Then I began calling printers in the phone book until I found one who seemed to understand what I wanted. He laughed when he caught on to my idea and agreed to help me. He thought it would make a good gift for some of his family, too.

Eagerly, I called a cab to pick up my written pages to deliver to the printer. I did not realize the stir it would cause at the nurses station when the cab driver arrived and asked for directions to my room. I chuckled when the head nurse burst into my room unable to believe that I had called a cab when I couldn't even sit up.

I called a special friend, Shirley, and asked her to bring me some pebbles. When I got them I borrowed some scissors from the nurse and cut out little pieces of my lamb's wool mattress pad and glued them to the tops of the pebbles so they had "fur."

Finally, the day came when the little booklet was finished. It included copyrights, a story, and several cute illustrations. It seemed to catch people's interest and they encouraged me to make it available in stores.

Several buyers I called agreed to place my pets for sale in their stores. Over the phone, I ordered little bags to put the pebbles and manual in so they made a "ready to send" gift. Calling my friend Shirley again, I asked if she would bring me some things not usually brought to patients in the hospital: a few yards of fuzzy material, electric scissors, glue, and a huge container of pebbles; she laughed but agreed.

It was evening before she could get there with everything. Shirley helped stretch out the material in front of me and I cut it into strips. She put the pebbles all around me in the bed so I could reach them, and hung the strips on the metal trapeze-pull-bar over my head until I cut them into squares to glue onto the pebbles. Since it was nighttime, I thought we would have privacy and be left alone to work.

Lost in the Hospital Bed

Unexpectedly, the door opened and there stood a new specialist who had come to examine me. It was obvious he was not happy with what he saw. As he tried to turn me over to look at my back, he grumbled that there were books, rocks, and little pieces of material all around me. The doctor complained that this was the first time he ever had a problem *finding* a patient in a hospital bed.

My face burned with embarrassment but it did not diminish my enthusiasm for my new project. Shirley couldn't keep from snickering at these circumstances and the doctor's surprised reactions. When he left, she continued to help me and then gathered up the finished little pebbles which had dropped all around on the floor.

The next day, I made arrangements for someone to deliver them to the stores for sale. Those first *Pebble Pets* sold out quickly, and the stores wanted more—a few hundred-dozen more.

I was thrilled! *Pedigreed Pet Pebbles*™ it seemed was a success. However, even when I offered to split the profits, I could not get ongoing help with this project. It was frustrating but I could not fill the orders. Shortly thereafter, *Pet Rocks,*™ a competitive product, came into the stores and I watched the sales figures climb out of sight.

Trying to console myself, I thought that maybe someday *Pedigreed Pet Pebbles*™ would be back. In the meantime, they would have to patiently wait to belong to their new owners.

My attention was once again focused on making it day by day and hour by hour. The pain in my back and down my legs was indescribable. However, I was determined to recover.

Logic vs. Faith

According to logic, reason, and medical science, I would never walk again; X-rays showed irreparable and permanent spinal damage. However, gradually and agonizingly, but miraculously, I forced, willed, and prayed movement and life into my back and legs. Bombarding my mind with positive suggestions—using *Sleep Learning* continuously in the hospital—I welded the words into my mind and heart, "I will, I can walk again."

My thoughts focused on faith-promoting slogans such as, "As you believe, so shall you receive. Set your mind on a course and watch the world step out of your way for its accomplishment" (Napoleon Hill). And I grew stronger every day.

I seldom read the newspapers that were brought each morning with my breakfast tray. However, this time, an article caught my attention. I showed the doctor the story about a lady who had an ankle injury for about three years and was healed in three weeks after using a *Transcutaneous Electrical Nerve Stimulation* (TENS) unit.

The TENS unit helps block some of the pain and promotes healing. The doctor ordered one immediately.

Slowly, I noticed a half an inch, then an inch of movement. With miracles, mental programming, and the use of the TENS unit to decrease the pain, I began making significant progress. Within ten days, I improved enough to be released from the hospital.

With a hospital bed in the living room of my house, I was able to go home. With the help of Mother and little granddaughter, I continued my recovery at home. Though my condition was improved and there was hope, I was still quite helpless; if the house had caught on fire, I could not have gotten out of bed by myself.

Mother had a full-time job but managed to assist me. After breakfast, she put things within my reach that I needed for the day. She put Crystal's and my lunch in the refrigerator and made sure the phone was near. She brought me a large drink, enough to last for the day. Then she left for work until evening.

My Little Angel

I don't know what I would have done without my mother's and granddaughter's help. Crystal was loving and sweet like a little angel. Having her there lifted my spirits and helped me in many ways. She was so cheerful and cute with her dark hair and beautiful large blue eyes; it seemed she was always smiling. We played school and sang songs. Then she would watch TV.

Prayer and Mental Pictures

With the bed piled high with the phone, books, positive mind-programming materials, and things for me to keep working on, I tried to generate some income. All materials had to be within arm's reach for me to use. Crystal would get things for me that fell. I kept the *Sleep Learning* recordings going continuously, programming my mind with the will and belief that I would accomplish my goals: I would walk again and succeed!

Living in a Spinning World

In early February of 1976, additional tests revealed I had an extreme infection between the discs that had not shown up in any of the previous tests. This was the source of my pain. It was called an *intervertebral disc space infection*. I was prescribed the antibiotic streptomycin.

However, a side effect and my body's reaction caused acute inner ear dysfunction, which resulted in the permanent inner ear damage with 100 percent loss of my balance (bi-labyrinthine dysfunction), which I still live with today. This added other challenges of living in a world that shakes and spins all the time because I have lost my sense of balance, gravity, and direction. I had taken for granted these marvelous systems of the body— until they were gone.

The First Law of Learning Is Repetition

Studying, pondering, and meditating on scriptures and books filled with Great Universal Truths, I programmed them into my mind and heart. Fervently praying for miracles, I remember meditating and mentally picturing creative ideas and opportunities coming into my life. I knew that thoughts are creative, and I mentally pictured miraculous results. I knew the first law of learning is repetition, and I kept repeating what I believed would work.

CHAPTER 14

Healing and Learning

In 1976, the United States and most of the Western world was in the midst of the energy crisis. The possible effects of the ongoing energy shortages had sparked widespread concern, and even fear. I too was becoming increasingly aware of the issues, and interested in finding answers to the problems.

I was interested in learning about and becoming more active in this area. I called schools, businesses, and governmental agencies for information explaining the problem and need for solutions.

A Business Idea

One day the phone rang. It was an acquaintance telling me he knew of a successful CEO who was knowledgeable in these subjects. He told me my questions could probably be answered by this gentleman and arranged a luncheon appointment for us. I had been careful not to let the seriousness or the after-effects of my surgery be known. I knew that feelings of pity for my situation would not attract opportunities to me. He didn't even suspect I was still lying helplessly in a hospital bed in my living room. The businessman's time was flexible; I made our appointment for three weeks later. In spite of my surgeries and physical handicaps, I was determined to go.

Determination Creates Results

Thoughts of that waiting appointment helped me try harder every day until I could lift my head, sit up, and then with the help of a tight back brace, get up and walk. Finally, approximately two months after my release from the hospital, I kept that appointment and made it out of the house. Forcing back the tears, I cinched up my back brace extra tight, wore a long dress to cover my leg brace, and used a walking stick.

The businessman sent his chauffeur who helped me down the walk to the limousine and drove me to the meeting. They had no idea I could not have driven myself there at that time.

As we sat eating lunch and discussing revolutionary ideas, I braced myself against the arm of the chair trying to ease my pain. My back brace was cinched up so tightly to help hold me up that it almost cut off my breath, but I managed to conceal my discomfort.

Along with the energy crisis and our nation's dependency on foreign oil, we discussed the critical environmental issues the world was facing at the time. What seemed most apparent to me at the time was the need for a technology to emerge that could create energy from waste materials. For some reason, the idea seemed so fascinating to me that I decided to devote myself to learning all that I could about alternative energy.

At that meeting, I learned about potential opportunities for women-owned firms in the field of environmental health. Creative ideas came into my mind that seemed workable. This opportunity seemed a tangible answer to my prayers. The businessman wished me luck on my new quest for further information and had his chauffeur drive me back home.

Keep On Keeping On

With new crutches, back braces, leg braces, and the medical TENS unit that sent electrical stimulation to my spine to help ease the pain, my travel and search for environmental solutions in the high-technology industry began.

With all I was learning about the need for and possibilities of alternative energy, I found a determination to do something about it. Forging ahead was not easy, but I felt I had to "keep on keeping on." During this period of time, however, I not only walked on my own, but traveled to many areas and met with many interesting and knowledgeable people. Pursuing my education, including specialized training, I learned about environmental health solutions for private industry and governmental agencies.

Later that year, my condition had improved greatly. The antibiotics helped the infection in my back which helped to relieve much of the pain.

The remaining pain I could mask. I also learned to adapt to my spinning world, and no longer needed the leg and foot braces.

Belief Leads to Action

In the late 1970s, I found it was difficult for women to be taken seriously in business. I made sure I maintained a professional persona. I used my maiden name and started J.E. Hunt & Associates for acquiring contracts for the engineering and construction of alternative energy projects and facilities.

I was able to arrange for a loan that I used to increase my education. I traveled to conferences and seminars across the U.S., from Chicago and Indiana to Kentucky and California, which opened the door for meetings with top scientists and engineers from around the world. Also, I received training as a professional consultant.

I still remember holding firmly to the following success formula:

$$Ingenuity + Courage + Work = Luck\ \&\ Opportunity$$
and that
$$Luck + Opportunity + Faith = Miracles.$$

With courage and grit, I started on a new adventure.

While working to obtain the sought-after contracts, I received many negative comments such as, "Why don't you go back to the kitchen and leave complicated things to men." And "Women were never meant to work in a man's world." And, "What makes you think you can do this? Women can't work in a man's field." Those comments hurt but did not deter me.

CHAPTER 15

Addiction, Antabuse, and Two Different Shoes

It was around this time, the late 1970s, that I was searching for a solution to the ongoing pain of the failed back surgeries. I finally went back to visit my physician. I told the doctor that I was still in a lot of pain and that the pain was distracting me from putting my full focus and energy into my business. My struggle was further compounded by insomnia, caused in part by the stress and pressure of competing in a male-dominated profession at a time when the majority of men, and many women too, frowned on women in business.

Unfortunately, after assuring me that there really was nothing more that could be done, the doctor made one other suggestion that turned out to be really bad advice. He suggested that I start drinking alcohol. "A little bit of wine," he said, could help to "dull the pain" and "soften the edge" of the relentless pressure and stress. The doctor also said that wine would help me sleep better.

What we now know, however, is that the sedative properties of alcohol may in fact help you *fall asleep* faster, but that, as your liver enzymes metabolize alcohol, the *quality* of your sleep is significantly disrupted. This can lead to excessive daytime sleepiness. Worse still, we also now know that alcohol can hinder your ability to retain what you learn for up to two full days.

Sadly, oblivious to these harms, I quickly took the doctor up on his suggestion. Without realizing how much alcohol was actually contributing to my daytime sleepiness, memory problems, and increasing stress, I simply decided to trust the good doctor and kick back with a couple glasses of wine.

Perhaps the real problem was that I was starting to enjoy the wine. And since he never actually defined "a little," and since my problems seemed to be getting worse, I decided to drink a little more wine. And then a little more. Before long I realized the wine was not enough. I don't think the doctor ever mentioned vodka, but since the alcohol was effecting my memory, I told myself that he never said wine, he said alcohol and, so, vodka must work just as well-only faster with fewer calories.

Within a few months I was drinking too much. I went from wine to vodka because it acted faster and stronger. I told myself it was dulling the pain, but even if it did make me more oblivious to the pain, it was creating other problems.

In retrospect, I knew I had a problem because I was trying to hide the fact that I was drinking every night. I don't know how many people I fooled, but probably not everyone. My mom certainly knew I had a drinking problem. But the problem was not the toll it was taking on my social life and relationships. The really big issue was how the constant drinking was effecting my brain. I started to forget basic things.

One day, my little drinking problem hit what I like to think of now as the bottom. I was attending an important electrical contractors meeting and I needed to be at the top of my game. Instead, I arrived still feeling the after effects of drinking the night before.

At first, I thought the meeting was going okay. That is until one of the men, stopped and pointed down at my shoes and asked, "Why are you wearing two completely different types of shoes?"

I looked down and was instantly mortified. I had been so impaired from the alcohol that I never even noticed. Perhaps, I could have blown it off with a witty reply. Instead, I immediately excused myself and rushed over to the table to sit down, with both of my legs tucked deeply under the long white tablecloth. When the first speaker went up to the stage, they dimmed the lights so we could see his slides. "This is my chance," I thought to myself. "If I walk out now no one else will know that I'm wearing two different shoes." I made it outside without anyone noticing. Minutes later, I was on my way home.

Unfortunately, I missed a few great speeches. I also missed the chance to make any meaningful connections with the other attendees.

Looking back, I realize this was not the sort of devastating bottom that all too many unfortunate alcoholics have to endure. Nevertheless, for me, this was a key turning point. I knew that my choice of shoes was due to the alcohol and I feared that others were going to find out that I was drinking. I was embarrassed and ashamed and, for the first time, I had to admit to myself that I had a problem with alcohol.

I made up my mind right then and there that I was going to quit—no matter what. I simply could not afford to have my judgment so impaired by alcohol. My dreams were at stake. Something had to be done.

I made a commitment to myself to quit, but I wanted to do something definitive, so that there was no other possibility. The following day I got a prescription for *antabuse*—which basically makes it impossible to drink without becoming violently ill, and which lasts up to 3 or 4 days. That was enough to do it. Never again did I struggle with the desire for a drink.

In the years since, I have sought to use my experience as a way to help others overcome their addictions. Whether it is drugs and alcohol, food, gambling, or sex, tens of millions of people struggle with addiction. If you include behavioral addictions, such as a compulsive or obsessive desire for shopping, gaming, pornography, texting, social media, and even work, the number of people struggling with addiction today is astronomical.

Whatever addiction you or someone you love may be struggling with, there are a number of steps you can take to help break the cycle. I continue to use most of the following steps in a program that I developed that has helped many people overcome a variety of addictions. I encourage you to follow these same steps. You don't have to be stuck. You don't have to struggle with addiction for years and years. You don't have to revisit the past to be free in the future. There are practical action steps you can start to take right now to conquer addiction once and for all.

1. Set a timeline for quitting and make preparations in advance to set yourself up for success. This includes removing the triggers that lead to addictive behaviors, but it may also include being careful about who you surround yourself with.

2. Build a support network for yourself by surrounding yourself with friends and loved ones who will be there to support you when you make the decision to quit.

3. Change your environment by removing any reminders of your addiction from your home and workplace. Don't hesitate to take

serious measures to make your home and work environment a safe haven, removing whatever temptation may be necessary.

4. Focus on resolving the underlying issue. Addictions are often the outward manifestation of an inner struggle or stress. If you can identify the source of your stress and resolve or eliminate it, you may also be able to reduce the grip of the addiction.

5. Your mindset can play a surprisingly powerful role. Stress is not always about what is happening to you, but, rather, how you are interpreting what is happening. Find a more positive, constructive, and empowering way to reinterpret or reframe what is happening and you might just find the stress begins to resolve. This is especially true if your new mindset or belief leads to new, positive actions and behaviors. Sometimes changing your mindset requires a more concerted effort, or the help of a therapist or coach. But if you persist you will find that it is possible to reprogram your subconscious mind.

6. Read or listen to positive affirmations. As I discussed in an earlier chapter, listening to audio recordings on affirmations is one of the core practices that changed by life. I particularly benefitted from listening to sleep learning affirmations every night. You can unleash the power of your unconscious with these powerful, positive affirmations which can also have a healing effect on your mind and body.

7. Practice prayer and meditation to help you stay focused and calm. Never hesitate to draw on the powers of heaven. Truly miraculous things can happen when you put your faith in God.

Converting Garbage to Electrical Energy

In the spring of 1978, a large U.S. county put out a request for a proposal to take them out of the garbage business. The county was handling about 500 tons a day of solid waste. I decided that I could put all the pieces together that it would take to create a winning bid.

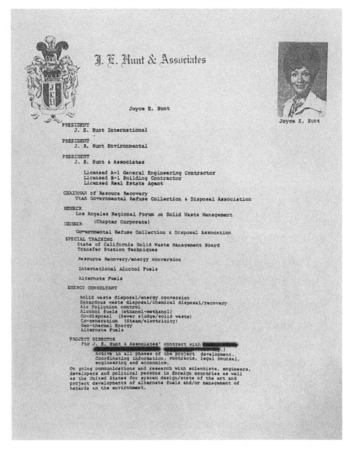

After additional intense study and hard work, at the age of 44, my efforts had paid off. Although several other companies, some that were well established, presented proposals, the one I put together was unanimously accepted.

I obtained a valuable twenty-year government contract. I was able to obtain marketing rights for a unique pollution-free patented process where we could convert non-recyclable waste to energy. I was also able to get my A-100 Engineering Contractor's license so I could build and own the resource energy and recovery plant.

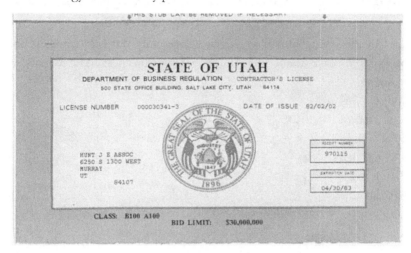

The future seemed secure for me and my family, and I was enthusiastic about it as I received recognition from experts in the fields of high-technology and environmental health.

This was a lucrative multi-million dollar recycling and waste-to-energy project. When it all came together, there were 35 employees and we processed approximately 500 tons a day of waste.

In this process, two pounds of garbage was equivalent to one pound of coal in BTU value. Our 500 tons of waste per day could produce enough electricity to light about 5,000 homes.

This was cutting-edge technology and over the next few years, top engineers came to tour our facility. Our hard work was paying off and we were fast getting ready to add the energy conversion to our recycling plant.

Contracts and Cash Flow

The project proceeded successfully beginning in 1978 and held even more promise as other communities requested similar contract information.

To simplify the day-to-day operations, I had entered into a contracted relationship with the division of a large, multi-billion dollar corporation. They agreed to provide me a percentage of the "net" profit if I allowed them to manage the overall project, including acting as project administrators and handling the accounting. And I relied on them. Together, we addressed the concerns of the employees, politicians, and the community. I worked hard coordinating engineering, organizing the projected construction, and arranging the financing.

My agents took charge of the cash flow and, at the time, I believed in their figures. Unfortunately, as much as I knew about the science and engineering aspects of the business, I mistakenly trusted them on the distribution of the revenues.

In our contract I had overlooked the precise wording. The contract provided that I would receive only a percentage of "net" revenues of the overall project, rather than a percentage of "gross" revenues. I never imagined the heart break and problems this single oversight would cause. I had trusted them only to find out later that they knew exactly what they were doing to me. There were always complicated excuses for why there was never much left over. I was under tremendous stress to keep the project running smoothly and "next year" was always promised for the project's "real" funds to be coming in that would benefit me and let my company develop as projected.

Since this one was coming along so successfully, they also encouraged me to travel to other locations to develop additional and similar projects all at my own expense. Believing my agents were taking care of things at the plant, I worked at becoming more knowledgeable in health concerns and in technology for the project's expansion. As I look back now, I can see they were hoping I would collapse under stress and financial strain.

Growing Expertise

In 1980, there became a great concern about a shortage of gasoline for our vehicles and interest turned to alcohol fuels. The debate back then was whether ethanol or methanol was better. Being interested in all types of alternative fuels, I attended a national conference in Ohio. The focus was on Bio-Mass to energy for use in cars. They called it Gas-Ahol, and most companies were focused on using corn. This brought me to my feet at the meeting and I stepped up to the microphone and said that we should be using all types of energy conversion to overcome our national fuel shortages. I also said that it's dangerous for the U.S. to be dependent on foreign oil. There are many waste products that could be converted to fuel.

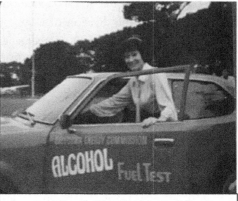

Joyce at the California Alcohol Fuel Conference.

Later, I was surprised to receive a Gas-Ahol news magazine with a picture of me at the microphone, with a comment below that read "it was pin-drop silence" as I addressed the six hundred, almost all male audience members who represented many companies and governmental agencies. My picture and statement was a full-page article.

Another conference I attended in 1980, was held in California. This was a three-day international alternative fuels conference. While there I became quite well acquainted with engineers from several other countries, including those from Japan, South Africa, Germany, England, and India. They were very interested in my project with its unique, cutting-edge technology. During our conversations, I was quite surprised to learn that some other countries were already using a variety of interesting energy conversion methods for bio-mass fuels. After further discussion, it became obvious that other nations were ahead of us in some of these areas and they wondered why the U.S. lagged behind.

Later, when I was back home, representatives from several municipalities and top companies in the U.S. contacted me. We met and discussed possible future projects in other areas needing to meet federal regulations for their waste disposal, as well as potential energy conversion plants.

A president of one of those large corporations invited me to Kentucky to meet with him and his top expert engineers who were involved in many areas of all types of energy conversion and hazardous waste disposal.

He picked me up at the airport and drove to his office in a high-rise building. I was a little surprised as we walked into his office and saw there was a chair for me directly in front of his four seated engineers. I felt like I was in court and the engineers were judges. Each engineer was an expert in a certain field.

Their demeanor was like, "Who is this woman and what does she really know?" They began to ask me questions about various topics such as federal regulations for ocean dumping and reclamation, landfill containment to protect soil, aquifers and water ways. They questioned me about air quality control and waste heat boilers, verses pyrolysis, and how the heat would create steam turbines to generate electricity.

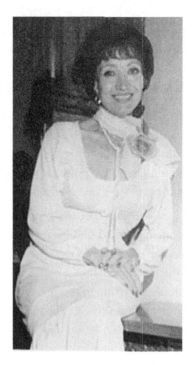

Joyce, as a businesswoman, in the summer of 1981

They questioned me about specific methods for coal gasification and a system that would extract oil from tar sand and oil shale. They questioned me about the feasibility of utilizing geo-thermal energy, explicit techniques concerning environmentally safe methods for hazardous waste disposal, and more in-depth questions about co-disposal of sewage sludge and solid waste, as well as the co-generation of steam and electricity without the use of fossil fuels.

Finally, after about three and a half hours, they took a break and said they would get back with me shortly. Within twenty minutes the president came back in, pulled a chair up beside me, and said, "Joyce, do you realize you're at least ten years ahead of anyone in our company. We look forward to working with you on a project."

After a few days of arriving back home, I received an official letter from them stating they recognized my expertise in the fields we had discussed of co-disposal, alternative energy and more. The president confirmed they were looking forward to working with me on a future project. Unfortunately, and unexpectedly, my circumstances changed and I was unable to follow up on these additional opportunities.

Gaining Knowledge and Confidence

By this time, I had regained my health to a remarkable degree. Now, no one could tell by my outward appearance that I still had a lot of back pain and problems with my balance. I had worked at concealing these conditions to the point that it was extremely difficult for me to admit that I had pain or needed medical care.

Knowing this, my physician gave me a letter to carry when I traveled explaining that I understate my problems with pain. Also, because of having severe labyrinthine dysfunction (balance problems) he gave me a letter which explained that I was not precluded from driving, even though walking was difficult for me. (I still carry up-dated letters in case of an emergency.)

When I was able, I attended international business conferences and gained valuable knowledge as I studied advanced technology and went to specialized seminars. It was fascinating listening to and interacting with top scientists from all over the world as they discussed solutions to environmental health and hazard problems.

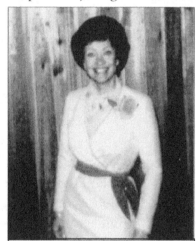

Dr. Joyce, President of J.E. Hunt & Associates

Opportunities were abundant to provide needed solutions working with some of the leading engineers in the world. With a team of knowledgeable and professional experts from companies such as Dow Chemical Co. and E.F. Hutton, I was eager to develop other potential projects.

Part Two

My Experience
in the
Spirit World

CHAPTER 17

Skull Fracture

One night in December 1981, I awakened with a stabbing pain in my right eye. A dim nightlight cast the only glow in my dark bedroom. As I was getting up to find out what was wrong with my eye, I found that my leg muscles wouldn't support me. In the near-darkness, I lost my balance and fell. My face struck something on the floor that fractured my skull in two places around my left eye socket. However, my attention was predominately on the pain in my right eye. It felt as though a large foreign object of some kind were in it.

The next morning, I went to an ophthalmologist. After examining my eye, the doctor put a patch over it saying I had scratched the cornea. He said he would not know for ten days whether I would lose the vision in it. X-rays showed the skull fractures. Nothing could be done for the swelling and fractures around the left eye.

Hardly believing this was happening to me, I nervously laughed when I looked in the mirror at myself with a swollen, black eye on the left and a big patch on the right. It became even more of a struggle to be positive and to avoid feeling sorry for myself. My eye issue was a scratched cornea, but the sight in my other eye was also threatened, due to my skull fracture.

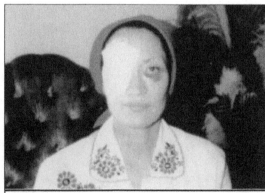

Joyce when she had a skull fracture and a scratched cornea (she almost lost her eye).

After a few days I recovered somewhat, and continued to keep in regular contact on the phone from my home office. No one on the project or my other associates were aware that I was injured.

I was able to coordinate final engineering construction and financing while using the phone for the 30 million-dollar energy conversion plant. In designing this project, I worked with top engineers from all over the globe, but especially with world-renowned engineer Ellis Armstrong, who served as the U.S. Commissioner of the U.S. Bureau of Public Roads from 1958 to 1961, and the U.S. Commissioner of the Bureau of Reclamation from 1969 to 1973. Armstrong was also the former Chairman of the World Energy Conference, and he oversaw the early development of President Dwight Eisenhower's Interstate Highway System.

The assigned agent from the large company I had contracted with who was supposed to be working for and on my behalf on my energy conversion project, would call me and come up with multiple reasons why I should not attend our monthly meetings with representatives from the county and the employees.

Gradually, I felt intimidated by their put-downs and sly comments. Perhaps I wasn't needed at the meetings anyway. The contract was definitely in my name and they told me I had nothing to worry about.

From the way they treated me, it became difficult to even be around them. Not realizing it at the time, with their subtle pressure and intimidation, I was developing a severe condition known as agoraphobia. It progressed to the point where I didn't want to leave the house and was reluctant to even be in small crowds.

Unbeknownst to me, the multi-billion dollar company that I had legally contracted with to work for me, used the time that I was not physically present, to advance their agenda of replacing my contract with their own.

The business was doing very well, but somehow my percentage of the profit was always small and was not covering my expenses.

Pushed to the Edge

I was assured by my agents that my presence was not needed at the project. A bleak and lonely Christmas came and went while I was not only house-bound with pain, but worried that I might be losing my vision.

On New Year's Eve, I was still confined to the house, not at all happy with what was going on. That evening, I was sitting in my living room pondering my situation, feeling sad that I had missed all the possible fun of the holidays.

Feeling water dripping on me, I looked up and saw the ceiling over my head sagging. With a shock I realized that the roof was leaking. There was so much water damage it actually almost caved in. I had replaced the roof only three years before—an expensive, messy job I didn't want to go through all over again.

Everything seemed to be pushing in on me at once: my loneliness, the stress associated with my business and lack of money, the severe pain in my back, the possible loss of my vision, and now the leaking roof. I sat in the chair pondering the many problems that weighed on me while I watched the water falling on the furniture. My habit of thinking I wanted to escape my Earthly challenges resurfaced as I thought, "Oh, let me out of here; I want to die. I just want to die."

In January 1982, while I was still recovering and dealing with all the business and personal issues and expenses, I fell again. I went down hard and broke bones in two places, my lower back and tail bone. It hurt terribly. (It was not until years later that I learned that my muscle weakness that caused my falls was an early sign of ALS, a progressive neurodegenerative disease, also known as Lou Gehrig's disease.)

Respiratory infections began plaguing me, and I was frequently bedridden with one illness after another. I would get a sore throat and be unable to get over it. The doctors weren't sure what to do as I began having severe reactions to the prescribed antibiotics. I began hurting and aching all over. My muscles were weak and I had trouble swallowing. If I cannot get well, I thought again, I just want to die.

With all of this weighing down on me, my thoughts went to when my father committed suicide in 1980. I remember there were only a few people at his grave-side service. I listened as they discussed my father. They talked about how he had a successful detective agency, bought and sold real estate, and was a commercial building contractor of shopping malls and housing developments. I remember them saying how brilliant he was.

They discussed how he had become very wealthy with these businesses, but had a recent huge loss which was apparently so overwhelming, that it contributed to his decision to commit suicide. I had sat staring at his steel, gray casket, vividly thinking that death could be the answer for me too.

Now, my leaking roof, recent fall, and my own financial and health situations brought back to the surface my own thoughts of wanting to die again. Later, I learned these were some of my better days for a long time to come!

Wanting Peace in a Beautiful Place

Believing in God and Heaven, I wanted to go to that beautiful place and have the peace of mind I had heard others tell about. I began praying that I would die. As time passed, I became physically worse with episodes of intense sweating followed by intense chilling. Also, I developed an allergic reaction to the chemicals in my clothing. In fact, many items in my environment that had never bothered me before would trigger a series of sweatings that would leave me drenched, and then I would chill.

Many days Mother came to take care of me. To battle the sweating and chilling, I changed my clothes several times a day. It took much of my strength, along with her help, for me to have dry clothes—and to just exist. Some special friends and neighbors often shopped for me and brought in meals.

Striving to overcome these ailments, I wanted to believe that any day things would get better. I wanted to conceal my illness. I had been assured by my agents that they were competently working in my behalf and that I was being properly represented at all meetings; I was told that my presence was not necessary. Not feeling needed by anyone, I avoided contact with friends and associates except for phone calls when I was feeling well enough to talk.

My condition fluctuated, but I became progressively worse. The doctors couldn't tell me what was wrong without running extensive tests. Since I no longer had insurance, I could not afford the tests.

In mid-1982, I contracted pneumonia and upper respiratory infections and became allergic to the antibiotics. In addition, I was diagnosed with rheumatoid arthritis. I grew weaker, was in constant pain, and became bedridden. Again, I just wanted to die.

Give Me This Day . . . Lasting Peace in Death

As the pain became more severe, I began asking caring friends to pray with me that I could die and be released from these trials. They told me they were praying for God's will to be done. They also said that as they prayed they felt that I was going through these trials for a purpose, but that I would have my choice to live or die. I had made my choice. I wanted to die!

The bronchitis and respiratory infections continued. Then I began bleeding from up inside my head and down my throat. I would wake up in the mornings almost unable to breathe. Consulting an ear, nose, and throat specialist, X-rays showed no medical problems, and the doctor could not pinpoint any cause for my problems.

A whole year had gone by since I started this downward spiral. It was December 1982 and I was still painfully alive. Believing that my family didn't really need me anymore, I continued to wish I could die naturally and be released from this living hell called life. The pain in my joints and body increased, and I could walk only by bracing myself on furniture.

Ticket to Paradise

When I was 49 years old, in January 1983, being still so ill and in so much pain, a doctor I greatly respected performed some extensive tests. Afterward he told me that I had an extremely low white blood cell count, so I was not fighting off the repeated pneumonia; I would continue to get worse. My body's ability to heal was failing, and there was no hope for my recovery. I was bedridden with worsening rheumatoid arthritis. I would get pneumonia again and die a natural death in a short time.

On the day I heard this news, I believed God was handing me my ticket to paradise. I wouldn't have to commit suicide—I thought I would just die. With this news, I was sincerely more thrilled than someone would be if they had a winning lottery ticket. I was not going to have to end my life myself. I was just going to die and go to that place of peace that I wanted from the time I was a small child.

It was physically difficult that day to take my shower; but feeling so elated about dying gave me a little extra energy. I was fantastically happy that I was going to die and go to my imagined place of "forever happiness and joy." As the water sprayed over me, I was thinking of how wonderful I was going to feel when I left all my problems behind.

A song joyfully came to my mind and I sang parts of it: Somewhere over the rainbow . . . where troubles melt like lemon drops, away above the chimney tops, that's where you'll find me. The words and melody of that tune stayed in my mind for hours and lulled me to sleep that night with pleasant thoughts of my coming "trip." Those words portrayed the new attitude I had for the next few days.

My dying, I thought, would take a little time and that was okay! It meant I would be able to complete my Earthly affairs, such as making my burial arrangements. I would have to do them slowly because I was so ill. Still, I wouldn't leave my family in chaos, and that was important to me. I believed it would be much better for my loved ones when I died.

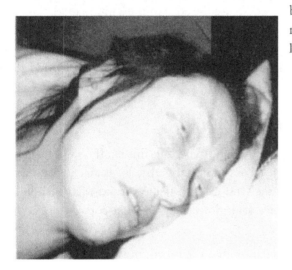

Snapshot taken by Crystal, my granddaughter, a few days before I went to the Other Side—January, 1983

CHAPTER 18

Entering the Spirit World

A few days later, I felt weaker and more ill than ever. I was alone that day. As the morning wore on, I continued to feel much worse. I began worrying and thought, I can't die yet; I'm not quite ready.

I wanted to pray, but was too weak to kneel on my own. The bathroom was large and attractive with an ivory-marbled tub and white-lace shower curtains. I decided I would use the edge of the bathtub to lean on. I managed to get into the bathroom even though the pain in my body was intense, and I had lost most of my strength. Supporting myself by leaning over the side of the tub, I maintained as reverent a posture as I could to pray.

I Wanted to Die—But Not Yet

I wanted to pray for just enough strength to finish a few critical tasks before I died. I bowed my head in prayer but before I was able to formally ask, I heard a voice as distinct and clear as if the speaker were standing directly above me. The voice said, powerfully, "If you come, you come now!"

With that, my strength left me and I slumped forward. All the air went out of me as I felt a sinking heaviness in my body. With a swoosh up and outward, I left my body and found myself behind and slightly elevated from my body, my feet not touching the floor. I felt weightless and all my physical pain completely vanished.

Spiritual Shock

I had thought that when people die, they went through a tunnel away from the world with its challenges and its problems to the beautiful, happy place I'd heard about— but I did not. I was shocked that death and dying was not what I had expected it to be. The room seemed to have no limitations to my view as I looked up, around, and then down. Looking down, my attention focused on my body slumped lifelessly over the tub.

Immediately, I noticed the difference between seeing myself from the mirror's flat surface to observing my body's shape as another person could see it including a total view from the back. Looking around, I realized that my sight was not limited to the use of my eyes. I could see 360 degrees around me. I had always thought of vision as occurring in the one direction I focused on. But I could see behind me and in front as well as above me. In this sphere, there was sort of an instant visual awareness of everything around me.

I felt wispy, almost transparent. I was aware that I could go through a wall and my hand could go through anything. I was also very aware of my limitations without my body; the knowledge was simply there. Anything I had not said while on Earth would remain unsaid, anything I had not written while on the Earth would not be written. I could not pick up anything—not even a piece of paper.

Heavenly Hologram

It is difficult to describe what happened next. Events did not slowly progress from one phase to another as they had when I was alive on Earth. Everything seemed to be happening almost instantaneously. Consequently, it is difficult to separate this experience into periods of time or to differentiate it into stages. The Other Side's dimension and my experiences there were as a whole, like a hologram. God's universe is complete; it was magnificent beyond belief and absolutely beyond Earthly description. I saw that we are all connected and there is a reason for everything, even the fly.

Vast knowledge and immeasurably deep feelings relating to my own personal development accompanied everything I experienced on the Other Side. This was the most vivid, personal experience I have ever known. I have struggled to find the right words to share this marvelous, yet extremely anguishing experience.

The Spirit World Is Real

Vividly aware I was in a spiritual realm, I knew I was in a sphere of afterlife, a place without my body, a space and time before resurrection. I had not realized there were distinct phases of afterlife—the spirit world when I would be *without* my body, and resurrection when my spirit and body would be reunited.

This different realm was more realistic, authentic, and factual to me than Earth-life's sphere. This was, without question, the most stark, real thing I had ever experienced. All else seemed insignificant in comparison; but I was shocked that nothing in the spirit world was as I expected it to be.

Everything fit with a sharp reality, however, and with new knowledge in my mind. I had read in the Bible that the spirits of some people who had died long before Christ's resurrection were finally reunited with their bodies after *His* resurrection. I realized that they must have been in a wispy, spirit world similar to this one until the time of their resurrection.

A desperate longing for my physical body overwhelmed me as I realized how terribly limited I was without it. I wanted to communicate with my family, to tell them I loved them and missed them, but I could not.

My chance on Earth was over, and now it was too late. I realized with feelings of remorse that what I had thought of as dying and being in a state of "paradise" was not at all as I had anticipated.

CHAPTER 19

In the Presence of God's Light and Love

Suddenly, I was in the presence of God's Light and Love, an overpoweringly brilliant white light. I knew that my natural eyes could not have endured this light. His Presence was brighter than anything I could have imagined. He was glorious and inspiring—radiant with love. I was filled with an awesome knowledge about God, His power, and His love. It permeated my whole being, and I received my own special witness that Jesus is Christ, the Son of God, and He is filled with saving grace.

My belief in God was replaced with an absolute *knowing* that He is real! I know from my own personal experience that the Scriptures are true and that God is filled with Love, Mercy, and Grace for us all. As I learned on the Other Side, this is true regardless of the name or title people use to refer to Him. Whether people call Him "Creator of the Universe," "Higher Power," "Lord," "God," or "Jesus," His answer to me and to all of us is: "**I Am Who I Am.**"

There are many different religious teachings and faiths in the world. I suggest you keep looking until you know in your heart and soul, including through prayer, that you have found the truth of God.

How humbling! I felt I should bow or kneel to show my reverence. I had always loved my Creator, but I had never felt an actual personal relationship with Him.

While in His Presence, I was instantly and keenly aware of the fact that ***God is REAL!*** I was also keenly aware of a definite purpose for life. New understandings and meanings of life's happenings flooded my mind. And I knew that Earth life is the time to repent and prepare to meet God. *I was given heavenly answers for Earthly challenges.*

While on the Other Side, I was shown the importance of the Sermon on the Mount, and, as it says, "Blessed are the peace makers: for they shall be called the children of God." (Matthew 5:9, KJV)

I also learned the value of just listening, without judgment or providing a solution. Many people just need to talk and feel validated as someone listens. Whether they are right or wrong, they don't always want a solution, but just need to talk to someone and feel like someone cares. When we pray and tell our problems to God, He is an understanding listener. But we must also express gratitude and appreciation for the blessings we already have, and, in doing so, we may receive many miracles which we would not have otherwise received.

Whenever we feel a prompting, we should follow through, which could be for our own good, or others. Often, we could be the answer to someone's prayer. God usually answers our prayers through other people. We are more apt to have our own answers to prayers when we help others. For as we give, so shall we receive. Even if it's in the afterlife.

I felt horrendous regret for wasting so much valuable and limited Earth time, wanting to give up rather than learning and growing as I made it through life's problems and challenges. I essentially went through life with the attitude of a quitter. I lacked faith in a reason for living. Even though I understood the power of positive thinking, I didn't understand just how powerful our thinking is, or just how much our beliefs and our faith in God work together to create miracles. I had also bought into the popular myth that, just by dying, I would automatically receive an *unearned* peace. In other words, by lacking an eternal perspective, rather than realizing an *earned* peace and joy, I had brought on much of my own mental anguish and despair by my negative thinking and desire to give up.

Another great truth crashed in on me; had I died by my own hand, it would have caused great anguish to my loved ones and additional regret for me on the Other Side.

Suddenly, I heard a chorus of voices from those in the Spirit World who wanted to comfort their loved ones left behind on Earth, and especially those who were excessively grieving. They wanted to tell them that they are now their spiritual cheerleaders from the Other Side, to have faith, that God is real, and to move on with their lives and make the best use of their own limited Earth time.

God's Love

My love for God was greater than I had thought possible, beyond my Earth-life's comprehension. I realized God loved me unconditionally and that He knew all about me. My own self-awareness of my thoughts and actions was sharply intensified. I felt great anguish, remorse, and sorrow for things I had done in life that I knew I should not have done, and for things I knew I ought to have done that I did not do while I was alive on Earth. I wanted to shrink away from God and His Presence of love and truth.

As my understanding increased, my love for the Creator of the universe increased. I felt an overwhelming appreciation for the blessings I had received in life. However, the more that I realized the opportunities I had in life, the more my anguish intensified for having not used my time on Earth better.

The Being of Light standing before me radiated such a bright light it was difficult to make out particular features. But He was powerful, all knowing, and so loving. I felt His unconditional love radiating throughout my mind and soul. I had no idea there could be so much love for or from anyone, or that I had the ability to have these deep feelings of love for someone else. Instantly, I knew that people do not have to be in a high-ranking position in life for God to love them. His love is boundless, limitless. He loves everyone, and I realized how important all of us are to Him.

I thought of loving someone with an intense and all encompassing emotion, the most love anyone could ever feel for a child or a companion, and I knew that love is nothing compared to the love we have for our Creator as we come to know Him.

The Ultimate Joy—Being in His Presence

My earlier thinking was that if I could have a moment with God, or someone representing Him, there would be many questions I would like to ask. But I discovered I didn't desire to ask Him anything. I just wanted to enjoy His presence, to bask in His love, to be with Him.

Then I thought about being reunited with loved ones after a long separation. All I would want is to be in their presence, to love them, to feel their love for me in return. Bringing them up to date on events or quizzing them would seem pointless.

Feeling encircled in this love was a wondrous experience. I knew that the most horrible thing that could ever happen to me, my family, friends, or any of us who knew God would be to do something that would cut us off from His Presence. To be anywhere else but in that presence would truly be hell.

With new-found understanding of God's love, I knew I had let Him down. As I realized this, my understanding was opened. Knowledge flooded my consciousness and thousands of different subjects instantaneously lit up my comprehension. This experience simply defies explanation.

Inner Awakening

It wasn't that this knowledge was coming from an outward source—it was as though knowledge which had always been within me was awakened. It was as if, in an instant, a cloud evaporated from my mind and I had access to more knowledge and understanding than I had ever imagined. I knew my Creator was all knowing, all powerful, and able to reveal all needed things to my view.

In Scriptures and Holy Writings many great truths are taught in metaphors and parables; perhaps some of the things I was shown were visual parables of great truths. I saw things I was familiar with used as representations of concepts. I saw these concepts as complete blocks, not merely as words. Words were not necessary and thoughts were simply known and didn't need to be spoken.

Pure and higher forms of communication took place there—mostly through thoughts. By comparison, Earth-life communications seemed limiting and archaic. The free flow of ideas and instant understanding were so much quicker and clearer in the spirit realm. It was communication from mind to mind, being to being.

God-Given Answers

Always-present knowledge, Eternal Truth that in some way constantly surrounds us, was revealed to me. I understood that many of these Eternal

Truths are also available during life on Earth, although they are not easily perceived. They are available when the time is right and an individual is willing to make a deliberate effort to tune into the right wavelength. I was filled with a stark reality of knowledge. I discovered there is no new truth. Truth is eternal and ever-present.

Suddenly, the answers to questions and challenges I had in life came so quickly and seemed so obvious, I felt repentant for even wondering. I understood reasons for problems and answers to problems. I immediately yearned to go back to my life on Earth and share what I had learned with my family, loved ones, and others.

Sands in an Hour Glass

Also, I was aware I had created an anguishing hell for myself, because I could have done more with my time on Earth than I did. I knew that time, as it was known on Earth, was limited, running out like sands in an hour glass beginning at birth and continuing until death. Time was to be used wisely and however it was spent, it could not be called back. Earth life was the foreign sphere, and time on Earth was temporary, limited, and precious!

In addition, I became aware that our time begins counting down the day we are born. None of us know when our time will be over, not the day or the hour.

All that mattered, I discovered, was what I did with the opportunities I had, and I was not measured against what I did not have or what anyone else did or did not do.

Thinking of some of the people I had known in my life who had wasted a lot of their time hurting others, I realized that God sorrowed when they did wrong, but He still loved them. Feeling great sadness for them, I realized how they were really hurting themselves. I understood that each person has a definite purpose for living and only so much Earth time to fulfill that purpose.

Challenges and Rewards

Viewing my own life's experiences, I saw that learning self-control is a great challenge and takes time. Some of the greatest strengths we can develop are those required to control feelings and emotions, *especially the strength required to harness the tongue.* However, I saw rich, eternal rewards such as better family relationships that could be reaped by striving to master these things.

I knew that every act of kindness carries a reward. It was amazing to me that *even little kind acts could reap very large rewards.* Every good attitude, everything right I had ever done in my physical body had been a gift to God and to me.

My new understanding included knowing that any wrong deed I had done with unrighteous motivation or intention was actually hurting *me.* Many rewards that could have been mine were lost because of my own actions or my sins of omission. I was shown how everything I did during my Earth life had consequences; every action I took had a definite reaction and brought an appropriate reward or a just punishment—a cause and effect, as if I were planting seeds and reaping exactly what I sowed.

Planting and Reaping

Scenes flashed quickly before my view and I saw farmers of all eras—weary, medieval peasants tilling the ground with crude stick-tools, others dragging wooden plows; then futuristic, sophisticated machines crawling over immense fields, row after row, field after field, planting seeds. My interest and attention was not on the farmers or their surroundings; I was fascinated with the seeds and the miracles of growth connected to them.

Time was compressed. No sooner had they planted than they began harvesting what they had sown. Those who planted corn reaped corn, those who planted carrots reaped carrots. Those who planted rice reaped rice. Someone planting carrots would not reap apples. Whatever was planted was harvested—in its own kind.

This Life Is the Time to Plant

Rapidly, these scenes appeared to my view. Then the scenes changed, and now people were harvesting love and kindness because they had sown love and kindness with their intended actions, while beside them others were reaping hateful, hurt feelings and violence, because they had sown hate and hurting of others with their intent and actions.

Every kindness, every right decision, every forbearance was returned in kind; every cruel act, every hurtful decision, every quick-tempered retort reaped a like result. All the time these scenes were playing before my view, I recalled a proverb I had heard during Earth life: *As ye sow, so shall ye reap.* (Galatians 6:7)

The messages of the scenes I viewed became clear to me: forgiveness reaps forgiveness, mercy reaps mercy, love reaps love, violence reaps violence—the harvest of anger at others is anger directed at oneself. The eternal truth is that no one can escape harvesting what they plant.

Then I knew that Earth life is a time to plant, and the Other Side is the ultimate time of the law of the harvest— as we give, so shall we reap. I was reaping anguish because of what I had sown during my Earth life. I had made my own choices in life as to how to think and act. With my thoughts, actions, and *reactions* to situations and to others' actions I had created for myself what I was receiving. I had not realized that while I was alive on Earth I had been building my character, my spiritual being, and determining my own harvest of eternal rewards, or lack thereof. I discovered that I *chose* joy or agony by my thoughts and actions during my Earth life.

Also, I had a vivid awareness that studying Scriptures and Holy Writings would have revealed great truths that were grand keys to solving problems, achieving lasting peace of mind and eternal enjoyment.

During my Earth life, my love and knowledge of the Great Creator of the Universe was limited, but now I was filled with His love for me and mine for Him. My love and gratitude to Him for my many blessings seemed endless; my love for others was increased—it was all-encompassing—and I realized how important we all are to each other. Again, I was filled with anguish for not having used my time on Earth more productively. I had wasted precious time wanting to die. Being in God's presence made me wish I had used every minute I had on Earth planting love so I could reap blessings.

CHAPTER 20

A Spirit Contorted in Sorrow and Pain

Suddenly, I seemed to be transported through time with scenes quickly passing my view. Then I was in a chapel with flowers everywhere—large beautiful bouquets on pedestals. The room was crowded with somber people; the only sounds were soft whispers and muffled sobbing. I could see everyone there, but they could not see me and no one reacted to my presence.

Glancing around, I saw a line of mourners filing slowly past a modest casket. The body of a young woman with shoulder-length, strawberry-blond hair was lying in the casket. Mortuary skills and cosmetics had given her a placid expression; she looked peaceful and beautiful. How sad, I thought—such a young woman robbed of everything Earth life had to offer.

My view then focused on an older woman sitting off to one side. She seemed dazed, her eyes staring into space. The pain emanating from her was undeniable. I knew at once she was the dead woman's mother, hurting as any parent would when burying one's child. Two beautiful little girls, perhaps four and six years of age, were with her. They were daughters of the deceased woman and this woman's grandchildren, and they were sobbing uncontrollably. Their hair had been lovingly done by a caring relative and they were both dressed in frilly, blue dresses with white lace trim.

Somehow, I knew these dresses had been purchased by their dear mother for a happy occasion in the recent past. Now they were being worn for her funeral. The youngest child sat on her grandmother's lap, clinging to her and weeping. The six-year-old stood at the side of the grandmother, her face buried in her hands. Her little shoulders shook with her sobs. The children could not stop crying, but their grandmother, in such pain she hardly seemed to realize they were there, was unable to offer comfort.

I understood her thoughts: How was she ever going to take the place of the children's dead mother? She was older, with few financial resources and even fewer physical resources on which to draw. How could she ever love them enough to ease the pain of losing a mother who had left them?

The Anguish of Reaching Out in Vain

The dead woman had not died in a tragic accident or of disease. This knowledge came vividly to my mind. She had taken her own life, died by her own actions, voluntarily giving up her chance to accomplish anything more during Earth life.

Suddenly, I saw the spirit of the young woman kneeling at her mother's feet. She was different from the others in the chapel. Her body was not full and solid as were the bodies of her mother and children and the other mourners. She was wispy and transparent as I was at that moment—a spiritual body, not a physical one—and her face showed sorrow and pain. Her mortal body lay a few feet away in the coffin, yet her essence, her spirit, her soul was here, sobbing at her mother's knees. I heard her thoughts, her words. She was sorry for what she had done. She ached for them and the pain they were experiencing.

She reached out, unable to touch them or to be felt by them. Her desperate attempts to make herself heard or understood failed utterly. She tried to take the oldest girl into her arms to comfort her; she wanted to console, to caress her children, but they didn't even know she was there.

I listened as she begged their forgiveness. She was desperate to make them understand, but they could not hear her words. All she could do was watch as they suffered. I realized she had been a single mother raising these little girls alone. The emotional and physical responsibilities had overwhelmed her; she had come to the point where she felt that her problems and pressures were too great to endure. She felt depressed and allowed her feelings of despondency to grow to the point that she mistakenly felt that release from life was her only solution.

The Tragedy of Death By Choice

She had committed suicide thinking she would find peace. Our Lord is filled with love, grace, and tender mercy.

The consequences of taking her own life were nothing at all like the peace she imagined. I could sense her agonized frustration—she was unable to communicate with or console her loved ones. She was utterly helpless to aid them in any way.

(In suicide, as in all things, only God can judge. Only God can know what consequences we must face for our actions. Only God can determine what hardship we must endure for our own highest and best good, and only He can love and support us and carry us all the way through.)

The Ripple Effect

I knew that it would, in time, be well with each one of them, including the mother. Ultimately, nothing can surpass the sweet, loving Spirit of Our Lord and I know He will be with all of them in their journey through life and on to eternity.

The analogy of a pebble thrown into a pond came to mind. The ripple that results expands outward and ultimately affects an area immeasurably larger than the size of the pebble itself; the ripple travels on and on. I understood that every action in life, especially suicide, affects so many people that its effect seems endless. The ripples—often more like tidal waves—caused by the deed roll outward, touching many lives.

My Personal Hell

Having willed myself to die, akin to suicide in my case, I knew that my inner hell would be viewing the loved ones I had left, witnessing the repercussions of my actions. Such thoughts stayed with me throughout my experience. It would be my own personal hell seeing and not being able to alleviate the sorrow that my actions caused. I was my own judge and was now judging from the Spirit World's all-seeing, all-knowing perspective.

The knowledge that I could have done better was agonizing. Seeing my attitudes and actions in the light of truth was misery to my soul. I yearned to warn my family and others of the regret and sorrow that I was experiencing. Intensely I wanted to return to my mortal life and again have the privilege of living in my physical body even with its pain and illnesses—even with the same conditions I had sought to escape for so many years.

The Tragedy of Teen-Age Suicide

As quickly as I grasped this, I was shown another scene. Again, I was at a funeral, viewing a person who was deceased. I was standing at the head and slightly behind a beautiful, very expensive casket made of rich rosewood. I knew that this entire funeral had been elaborately expensive and that the high cost of the funeral was an attempt of grieving parents to soothe their pain.

As I watched, again no one seemed aware of my presence. Before me stood four mortal beings and a spirit personage. I understood at once who each person was and what they were feeling. Standing next to me was the spirit personage of a young man. His form, like that of the young mother I had previously seen, was wispy, nearly transparent. He was a good-looking teenager with sandy-colored hair cut short. His natural intelligence was apparent.

Wanting to Make Contact

His physical body lay in the open casket directly in front of me. I looked from one to the other in amazement. In contrast to his spirit self, his mortal body was solid, still, and lifeless. Its facial features were peaceful, as if he merely slept.

His spirit body, in contrast, was trying to make contact, he was reaching out his insubstantial, wispy arms to his father who was gazing down at the body in the casket. His father's shoulders were stooped from almost unbearable sorrow, his face drawn, his eyes swollen from crying.

Somehow I knew many things about this man. He was close to retirement with limited financial resources. He had stretched himself beyond his means to make this funeral elaborate, using money from his retirement funds for this final farewell, sparing no expense in an attempt to ease his grief.

The father was speaking softly to two young men; I sensed that they were best friends of the boy. Handsome young men, they were intelligent, personable, and well dressed. I realized they were leaders in their classes at school and that they seemed perplexed.

Thoughts about Futility Are Futile

What impressed me as I focused on these two young men was the depth of depression and hopelessness they both had been feeling for some time. The death of the youth did not create, but simply brought to the surface, their feelings of futility—the same feelings the deceased boy had felt when he took his life. I had wasted a large portion of my life feeling the same way. I too had believed the myth that all you have to do is die to receive instant happiness and peace.

The father was telling the friends that his son had been a troubled boy with many problems. He looked down at his son's body and rested his hand on the edge of the casket as he said, "He's at peace now." This was what the mourning friends and family wanted to hear. These words eased their sorrow and made this loss easier to bear.

"No, Dad!" the boy's spirit cried out, "Stop! Don't tell them that. That's not what they need to hear!" I watched as his spirit tried to gain his father's attention, and with sadness I realized why he was trying so hard to communicate with his dad.

False Hope

The bereaved father continued talking about his son having gone to a better and happier place. He told them his son was free from the pain and depression he felt while alive. I realized the father's words that he wanted to believe were true gave feelings and thoughts of false hope to the two young friends that they could find peace if they, too, committed suicide.

For these boys, the father's words were an invitation to join their friend—a confirmation of what they *wanted* to be true. They wished to believe that their friend was finally at peace, was finally free from his problems and sadness. They hoped that they too could find that peace. The father's words of self-comfort reinforced that message.

But their friend was trying to communicate to them that suicide is not a path to peace. He could see the way his friends were feeling—the father could not. Each boy was struggling within, making the decision whether to continue in a life he felt was hopeless or to end his life and find this beckoning peace. The spirit boy tried to communicate with them and convince them not to believe what his father was saying. "My father is wrong. Suicide is not the answer," he kept saying. "Please, guys, you must make it through your problems!"

The Myth of "Peace through Suicide"

The father continued speaking about how his son had wanted peace and freedom from worldly cares and that now he had it. The son was trying to communicate with his father, and trying to warn his friends not to make the same mistake.

He had taken his own life, falsely believing that in death he would find happiness, peace, and contentment. Instead, he found that it wasn't only these two close friends that would be impacted by his actions.

Suicide Is NOT the Answer!

If one or both of these boys chose to die, there would be family, other friends, peers, and schoolmates affected. Even strangers who would hear about his death or read the obituaries might be influenced into thinking suicide was a solution. I saw how feelings of hopelessness could compound, affecting many people, sweeping onward relentlessly like waves driven by storms far across the ocean.

I felt sorrow for the boy who had given up his chance at life on Earth, sorrow for the friends who were seriously contemplating taking their own lives now too. I recognized how my own life fit a similar pattern. I felt regret for my own thoughts and actions. I was suddenly struck by the truth. I found myself repeating the words of the young man, "*Suicide is not the answer! Suicide is not the answer!*"

I realized that only God can judge. Only God knows the intent of the heart. Given that our Lord is filled with love, grace, and tender mercy, I believed that the young man would someday have peace, but at the time he was filled with regret.

The Race of Life

I was then shown how life is similar to a race that starts at birth, and that when I was on Earth I was one of the participants. I saw scenes of a race, and I was running with other runners along a designated course. Then thoughts came to my mind: what if somewhere in the course of the race, I decided I couldn't wait to get to the finish line? Maybe I was too tired to go on, or I felt the race was harder than I had anticipated. Would this justify my cutting across the field, running directly to the finish line, crossing it, then expecting to claim the rewards of a great victory?

What would I really have accomplished? Even if I might fool those who didn't see me cheat, did I think I could fool the judges? Did I think they might conveniently be looking away at the exact moment I took the shortcut? Or could I console myself with the wish that they loved me so much they would forgive me—that no consequences would flow from my fraudulent action?

Did I think I could still be a winner if I didn't *earn* the victory? I knew it would be an empty victory and, in reality, a defeat. Even if the judges forgave me, I would still know. How long would I carry my guilt and shame before I could forgive myself? Lastly, what of the others who witnessed my cheating and were influenced to also take the shortcut? Would I not hold a part of their guilt as well? I recognized that taking a shortcut in a race is symbolic of suicide.

No Competition

I discovered that life is precious and only if I explored it to its natural conclusion, could I have the peace of mind and victory I hoped to claim. Also, knowledge was given me that during my time on Earth, I was not competing with anyone but myself. I knew that the only approval I really needed was from that Great, Loving, all-knowing Being, the Creator of the Universe—and from within myself.

CHAPTER 21

A Lightning-Speed Life Review

As I was being shown things in the Spirit World, suddenly, with lightning speed, my whole life began unfolding before me. I felt again the emotions I experienced during the actual times I first lived them. I was aware of the overall circumstances, aware that I was now in a different time and spiritual domain than on Earth when they first took place. The people I saw in my life review were not wispy, as were the spirits I'd seen. They looked rounder, more solid and natural, as mortal beings.

Instead of the limited perspective I'd had on Earth, this experience encompassed the feelings and viewpoints of all those involved, including the Creator's. With this perspective came a stark, resounding realization: life had not been the way it was portrayed in movies, books, songs, or newspapers. Life had not been as I had perceived it at all!

A Reality Check

In the Spiritual Sphere, I had a new, sharp awareness of reality. My life review continued, bringing with it an awareness of the feelings and perspectives of those with whom I had associated throughout my life. I was aware of the way they felt about my actions and our interactions. The review was difficult but informative. I experienced many and varied emotions. I was amused to realize that many situations I had thought were serious at the time were really not serious at all. I felt sincere sadness when I revisited the points in my life where I could have done much better.

Although moving with incredible speed, as though someone had put my life review on superfast forward, I quickly discovered I could linger on any scene that caught my interest, re-experiencing it moment by moment if I desired. My life review was extremely enlightening and continued to be supplemented by a series of scenes that were allegories and parables—a unique teaching experience tailored to my particular needs.

In life, I had been argumentative, especially with my mother. The review revealed clearly how foolish and hurtful all arguments had been. Experiencing others' feelings as well as my own during turbulent episodes was a painful, humbling revelation.

Repentance: the Great Eraser

I was surprised when I realized that wrong deeds for which I had felt remorse and repented of were not in my life review. Those things were gone!

Vividly, however, I realized *I could have repented* for the wrong deeds I was still seeing, such as seeking revenge, being easily provoked, or doing things that worked against my own life's progression.

Most of all, my experience on the Other Side taught me that Earth life is a miraculous experience—a time to sow good deeds for glorious heavenly rewards.

CHAPTER 22

A Sphere with No Competition

Suddenly, everything I had learned and seen was surrounding me in this sphere of endlessness. I was aware again of the presence of the Being of Light and His love that continued to radiate and powerfully encircle me. I knew with all my heart that He loved me in spite of the mistakes I had made in my life. His love was complete, all-knowing, and unconditional.

A great question then emanated from Him to me so strongly that it completely penetrated my being. *"In life, what did you do with what you did have, not what you did not have?"* Rapidly, the question engulfed me, commanding an answer. All that mattered, I discovered, was what I did with the opportunities I had, and I was not measured against what I did not have or what anyone else did or did not do.

My Excuses Melt in the Light of Truth

I began answering defensively with reasons and excuses, as I had in life when I felt I was being called to task for failure to reach a goal. It was easy to find someone or something to blame for my failures. I could justify myself with reasons other than my own shortcomings for my actions, feelings, or failure to accomplish certain tasks.

I believed my excuses were good reasons to explain why I hadn't accomplished more: my difficult childhood, others getting in my way, my poor health, a broken home, my continual strife with my mother, lack of opportunities, and my growing family of children who held me back.

More excuses came welling up within me. If only I had been blessed with strong, supportive parents and raised in an atmosphere of love and acceptance. If I'd had a happy, successful marriage. If only I'd had more money.

I was stopped short in my thinking as I felt all my excuses melting in this Light of Truth. I felt the thoughts and words coming from this Being of

Love and Light. *"The question has nothing to do with what you did not have in life or with your burdens or faults or problems. But rather, in life, what did you do with what you did have?"*

All My Walls of Defense Melted

Oh, the humility and the guilt I felt at that moment. All of my life's actions were seen and known. I couldn't hide them or cover them and my carefully erected walls of excuses that had shielded me from accepting responsibility melted around me. All that was left was just me and the Being of Love and Light who knew everything about me.

I could not rely on or blame anyone else; this question was directed solely at me. I was being measured against no one else—I stood alone, on my own. What did I do with *my* life, with what I had, my opportunities, my time on Earth? *What had I done with what I **did** have?*

Suddenly I realized that difficulties during Earth life were really opportunities. I recognized how problems could be blessings when viewed from the Other Side.

Measured Against No One Else

On Earth the goal is to win; it is certainly the over-riding desire of sports teams. Winning is the measure of success during Earth life; winning means fame and money. Losers are remembered only if the circumstances are humorous, sad, or if the loss is embarrassingly big. The label of "Loser" is energetically avoided.

Competition is fierce in most aspects of mortal life— from entrance requirements to college to parking spaces at the shopping mall. I was amazed to realize that in the afterlife sphere there is no win or lose, no competition with anyone else. Only *what I did with what I had* mattered. What I did *not* have was irrelevant.

Doing the Best We Can with What We Have

If only I had known to teach my family to do the best they could without the emphasis on winning or losing—to pay attention to how they lived the game of life. Life actually is like a game in a way, but the score that matters is not determined by wins and losses according to the world's standard, but by doing the best we can with what we have.

I now understood that there was no real defeat on Earth—only my own choices of attitudes and actions mattered. The important thing was to have kept going, to have looked for solutions, to have striven and endured well until the end of life—to have desired and to have kept trying to live in harmony with Eternal Truths. I realized the need for everyone to help the world be a better place for those living, as well as for future generations.

The Torment of "If Onlys"

In many ways, what I had *not* done with my life seemed more significant than what I *had* done to this point. I knew that every day I had lived on Earth I had exchanged a day of my life's time for whatever I had chosen to do that day. Many days I had squandered my fortune of time and now I saw what I had thrown away.

I was very aware that there is eternal joy to be reaped from seeking to do kind deeds and from not being easily offended, on Earth and for eternity. I realized that we don't have to be perfect during Earth life; just sincerely caring and making an effort to become more loving, charitable, and forgiving—and less judgmental. The desires and intent of the heart are so significant.

Miracles—More than We Know

As I understood Earth-life's purpose from an eternal perspective, I became aware that miracles happened abundantly and more easily for those who believed in them. Also, I knew my station or level of life was not as important as the direction I was going, and whether or not I was moving toward eternal goals, appreciating opportunities, and striving to improve.

On the Other Side, I learned that *trying counts*, and all sincere efforts are recognized with accompanying just rewards. My life review showed me with complete clarity that every choice I had made in attitude, thought, or action had an inescapable wanted or unwanted consequence. I alone was responsible for what I had done with my life.

CHAPTER 23

Perspectives from the Other Side

Prior to being on the Other Side, I had not understood reasons for burdens and adversities. It seemed unfair that so many trials and problems brought so much grief during Earth life. I wondered why some people have such dreadful lives of hardship and others seem to have relatively few problems. I learned that the answers could not be seen by viewing a short period of time in one's life on Earth. But from the perspective of the Other Side, which included everyone's feelings and viewpoint—even the Creator's— everything fits together.

Rich rewards and priceless joy await humble people on Earth who valiantly suffer through their trials and tribulations.

Opportunities Are Limitless

Knowledge came to my mind about people who were born with less than I had. I understood that we are not born into equal situations but we all have many more opportunities than we realize. I then knew that many of those who seem to have little according to the world's standards have the opportunity of reaping great rewards on the Other Side.

To Receive Mercy . . .

I learned that adversities are opportunities for personal growth and development and come with built-in benefits that can be enjoyed endlessly. I discovered that justice during Earth life is usually found only in the dictionary. Almost everyone on Earth is seeking justice, but justice means differing things to different people. What is just to one person is unjust to another. On the Other Side, however, there is complete justice. I recognized how important mercy is and how much more it can be received when it is freely given.

Free-Will Choices and Their Consequences

I understood that God permits us to make our own choices concerning our attitudes, actions, and especially reactions. God does not force us to do what is right during Earth life, and we do not have the right to force someone else to do "right" or to make "right decisions;" Earth life is a time to learn from choices.

However, I realized that even though God is saddened when we make choices that bring heartache or grief to ourselves or others, He still safeguards our free will to make these decisions. I remembered times during my Earth life when I had blamed God for my circumstances and my unhappiness. With this new understanding and perspective, I knew that most of my experiences on Earth were the consequences of my choices or my family's choices. Regardless of the difficulties, I could triumph over them with lasting results on the Other Side.

If We Don't Repent . . .

My understanding was opened further as I understood some of the ways repentance works, and that just and terrible consequences may await on the Other Side for those who do not strive to use their Earth time wisely and repent of their wrongdoings. When someone intentionally wrongs another, what awaits them is a confrontation of their improper actions and a full realization of their guilt and their lost rewards. However, I discovered that blessings and joy can be received by taking the opportunity to repent and do differently while we are still alive on Earth.

Earth life, I found, is designed as a university, a school where we learn from our choices and our mortal experiences. I recognized that my most painful experiences taught me the most. It was enlightening to understand the bigger eternal picture—to know that I was not a victim of circumstances. I learned that I could control my attitude and ultimately, my heavenly rewards.

The Coin Analogy

Suddenly an analogy came to my mind about problems and the difficulty of seeing them from a proper perspective. I wanted to tell my loved ones about a coping technique I'd learned—putting an object the size of a quarter to one eye while closing the other and then to liken that object to a problem. It would be so close that they could only see the problem, or the object. Viewed in this manner, problems can become overwhelming and can conceal obvious solutions.

Next, I envisioned light beginning to appear around the edges of the object as the hand holding it moved slowly away from the eye. Soon the object was far enough away that the things around it could be seen in perspective according to how it fit in and influenced the rest of life. Solutions could now be seen that had been there all the time, but had been concealed, eclipsed by the problem when it was out of perspective.

Every problem has a solution, and God knows that solution. One of the grand and rewarding opportunities of life is to communicate with Him and learn the solutions to our problems. His Light and Truth can flow to us for guidance as we work through problems rather than giving up on them.

Symbolic Parables

Immediately, I recognized this as a visual, symbolic parable of my own life. Problems would have seemed less devastating to me if I had been able to stand back and view each one in its eternal perspective. Answers would have presented themselves. Solutions would have become more obvious.

I realized I *had* grown wiser as a result of my problems and Earthly trials. But I saw that I could have gotten through situations, problems, and crises easier and been much further ahead in life, if I had envisioned the end result of my actions instead of staying caught up in the problem.

A Bag Full of Problems

Then I thought of times I had looked at people who seemed problem-free. At times, I had even wished I could trade places with some of them and have the life of peace and ease I mistakenly thought they had.

In the Spirit sphere, a story I'd heard on Earth about comparing other people's problems to my own vividly came to my mind. My consciousness was filled with scenes of this visual parable. I saw myself sitting in a roomful of people who were successful and problem-free when measured by worldly standards.

We were passing around a large, dark-colored, expandable bag and all the people were stuffing their problems into it. I could see their trials and challenges that had previously been hidden from my view as they put them into the bag. I realized that if I'd really known these people, I'd have realized that they, too, had problems that seemed as difficult for them as my own did to me. Many of them had even more problems than I did.

As soon as everyone had placed their problems in the bag, it was tossed into the center of the room. The bag popped open and all the problems began spilling out.

Instantly, everyone scrambled to reclaim their own. I dashed in among them, suddenly desperate to find my own set of familiar problems and trials. I did not want anyone else's—only my own.

My Problems Were Tailor-Made Just for Me

I now realized my problems were my own personal, educational building blocks, tailored just for me. Learning from my problems—the cause and effect from my choices, and my parents', and their parents' choices could help me overcome undesired social, cultural, or unwanted family traditions.

Suddenly, I knew I would not want to trade places with anyone else. I needed to grow and develop in my own way, which was different than any other person's way. Someone else's life experiences would not help me to become the individual that I needed to be. I needed my own individualized training.

I now knew that facing challenges builds the "muscles and strengths" of spirit and mind. Only through such exercises could I have developed as I needed to do. To build physical muscles, we lift weights. To develop the "muscles" of mind and spirit, we have the chance to solve problems, grow wise through them, and gain skills, knowledge, and talents that remain with us forever.

People Are More Important Than Things

Great truths flooded into my mind. I understood that the more people learned and applied on Earth, the more advantage they gain on the Other Side. I realized that when I died, I left behind all material wealth and worldly goods. They didn't really matter anymore—people mattered. I had a vivid awareness of how important people are, especially one's own family.

With new, expanded knowledge, I also knew the importance of learning and developing skills of patience and communication with family and others in Earth life; there are endless benefits in the spiritual sphere. I learned that being charitable, patient, and forgiving toward others are some of the most important character traits to be acquired—learned from the school of life.

My perspective had changed completely. These scenes brought me priceless learning experiences, but my learning had just begun.

CHAPTER 24

Spiritual Muscle Builders and Coping Techniques

More thoughts came to my mind about lessons I'd learned from troublesome situations. I thought of times I wanted to stay on a plateau. I heard myself saying, "No more growth, God, please. Let me just stay where I am. Please let me rest through a nice coasting period." Instantly, I realized there's no such thing as coasting—I was either going forward in life acquiring good habits or I was going backward acquiring bad habits, such as being impatient or developing an "I don't care" attitude.

Opportunities for Growth Abound

Returning to scenes from my life review, I was struck with the realization that daily or routine tasks presented opportunities for strengthening personal characteristics of patience and understanding for others. Previously, when people did things I thought were rude—such as crowding in a ticket line or cutting in front of me in traffic—my desire for justice surfaced and I felt compelled to verbally express my views to them, whether they could hear me or not.

I watched many of my actions and *reactions*. Most of the time when I got behind the wheel to drive, I was in a hurry and thought of driving as going from point "A" to point "B." Anything that happened along the way to delay me from my goal aroused my anger.

However, when I observed these scenes from this new perspective, knowing my feelings and also many of the other people's feelings and attitudes, it suddenly seemed foolish and childish to react impulsively and point out others' faults on the highway or anyplace else. I no longer wanted to judge others' motives. I knew the drivers did not realize the full consequences of their actions, as I had not previously, and that impulsive actions could lead to deadly accidents with rippling effects that could cause great anguish.

Angels—the Unknown "Back-Seat Observers"

Driving a vehicle, I saw, was one of many routine tasks that present opportunities to develop good character traits. It was also a definite "mini-test" of character—of how we think, act, and *react* toward others when it *seems no one is watching* or when we think our actions are not really important. Driving in congested traffic can be a great opportunity to build patience.

All situations and challenges, I saw, can be learning experiences. I could have reaped benefits if, when faced with a challenge, I had asked myself, "What can I learn from this situation?" Also, I discovered that it had been a waste of time trying to wish away my challenges, problems, and trials; they were my "spiritual muscle builders."

The Hundred-Year Coping Technique

Coping techniques I could have used in my life became easier for me to understand. I saw that I could have taken a problem or a difficult situation and examined its significance one hundred years from now by asking myself:

Who would have been affected by it, and how? Given that much time, did it still seem major or was it now minor? Taking that problem and sending it one hundred years into the future, how big or how small did it become? Could I even see it? Did it really matter in the outcome of my life? Many of my problems would have shrunk immediately if I had envisioned them by means of that simple technique.

Trials Pass

Life comes in phases, I realized, and each phase seems to stretch out in Earth years feeling as if it will last forever— but it never does. *Earth time is not forever.* Situations come and go, and *trials pass.*

I thought again of the young woman and the teenage boy who had committed suicide. If they had waited, things may have improved for them. It was tragic that by not realizing this, they had both taken actions that had forever stopped their Earthly growth and regrettably stifled their spiritual life.

We Find What We Look For

My life review continued. I saw that I had received great blessings, more than I knew. I was surprised as I became aware of times my life and my children's lives had been spared, and I realized that everyone on Earth has many more blessings and miracles than they recognize at the time.

Repeatedly, I realized that things in my life could have been much worse than they had been. When I was caught up in what went wrong, I overlooked the things that went right and the many blessings I had received.

One fact became clear: *I found what I looked for.* I learned it is better to look for and find things that have gone right—the many blessings received. I saw that by acknowledging and expressing gratitude for blessings received, *even more would be given.* I realized that life and each day had been a gift—if only I had noticed.

The Real Test

Like a light suddenly going on, I understood that if problems could bring blessings and opportunities, then the real test in my life was the intent of my heart and whether or not I had the right attitude. Even in situations that had gone badly for me, I could have passed the test if I'd had good intentions and the right attitude.

It became obvious that there were many times in my life where I had succeeded—such as times I had held my tongue and not argued when someone was verbally venting their frustrations as if I had been the cause of their problem. Joyfully, I was aware of some other times that I had kept good thoughts and intentions when it was extremely difficult to do so.

Life Is Like a Game—
With the Score Revealed on the Other Side

I realized that living in the world and accepting the tests throughout life builds character for eternity. Life is somewhat like a game—only the score is actually kept more on the Other Side than on the Earth. When my life review showed that there were difficult tests in life I had passed, I was filled with joy.

As knowledge filled my mind, I knew that *each of my adversities carried with it a seed of opportunity* for growth and improvement. But I needed faith to recognize and continue with patience until the growth was realized. That was the challenge—to persist and look for the good.

On the Other Side, the definite realization came to me that I'd had more opportunities than I realized while I was alive and situations could have improved. Then I knew that where I had *been* in Earth life was not as important as the *direction* in which I had been going.

Problems Refine the Spirit

Also, I learned that problems can refine the spirit—as I said before, they are spiritual muscle builders. I realized that there are all kinds of coping techniques available on Earth if only we open our minds and hearts to them.

But now I believed it was too late for me to utilize the knowledge I gained for Earth life. *Being dead was so final!*

CHAPTER 25

People Skills Have Eternal Benefits

On Earth, my tremendous determination to push for fairness and justice in the world led me to have an argumentative attitude. On the Other Side, knowledge about communications and relationships poured into my consciousness. Scenes from eternity that I was shown seemed personalized for my instruction. Perhaps that is why I was shown many scenes about arguing, its futility, and the damage it causes to relationships

The Futility of Arguments

At one point in my experience on the Other Side, I saw couples involved in heated disputes shouting at each other. As I watched, I shared their thoughts, feelings, and emotions as they argued. It was almost as though I could step inside each person's mind and heart and know what they were experiencing.

Their Words Did Not Reflect Their Feelings

I was amazed as I observed what was happening: the words each person spoke were completely different from the feelings they had. It was clear that they did not know how to communicate what they felt toward each other or how to explain their feelings without verbally attacking the other person. Obviously they did not understand the other's viewpoint.

Also, what they wanted from their partner was not manifest in what they were saying. In fact, as they argued they strayed far from the original conflict. Their accusations became more outrageous, their demands more and more inappropriate, and they eventually resorted to name calling. However, each partner was feeling hurt and shocked that their loved one's words and responses were as unkind as their own.

One woman was spewing verbal threats at her mate, such as, "If you leave me, I'll take the children so far away you'll never see them again," and, "If you leave, I'll find someone so much better than you." But what she was actually thinking was that she loved her husband and wanted to put her arms around him and calm things for them both; she desperately wanted him to put his arms around her and tell her that he loved her. Not knowing her true feelings, he felt rejected and reacted to her words.

She didn't see that when she hurled angry words at him, she was sowing more anger. As certain as planted seeds yield their own kind, he responded to her hateful words with hateful words of his own—and she was hurt even more. His response was so different from what she wanted that she threw back even more bitter words and threats. The wrangling continued and pointlessly escalated. Their feelings were easy to perceive. They were both bewildered and wondered why the other person hurled back hurtful, vindictive words which surprised and further angered them.

As I shared their feelings, I knew that these arguments and angry emotions grew because of the frustration of not knowing what to say, what to do, or how to respond to the other's behavior. They simply did not know how to express themselves so the other person could understand their view point.

I knew that both the woman and her mate did not even mean the things they were saying; they reacted to what the other was saying without thinking of the consequences. They could not separate themselves from the contention long enough to act the way they wanted to, but trapped themselves in their arguments.

They each felt enormous heartache and emotional pain. I wanted to shout to them, to tell them to stop and listen to what they were saying. If one of them would take time to think about the situation and understand what the other was really feeling, they could have changed everything. If either one of them had stopped criticizing the other and stopped the attacks on the other's most vulnerable points, they could have stopped the argument and avoided irreparable damage to each other's feelings and their relationship.

I learned that most arguments are futile and come from limited understanding of others and from limited communication skills. If a situation could be viewed from all dimensions, including others' perspectives, and if people could control their words, arguments could dwindle or even cease. Sincere empathy and unconditional love would replace the inclination to argue or hurt another.

Opinions Need to Be Listened to—Not Challenged

I understood that things would have been different if any of the people I had seen fighting had simply been strong enough to compassionately look at the other and quietly listen and accept their partner's opinions without contradiction. They had their own opinions and were at their own level of growth. They each wanted understanding of their opinion—to be non-judgmentally heard, and to feel loved and accepted. They did not want someone telling them what to do and giving unasked-for solutions.

Each partner needed to see things from the other's point of view without criticizing and giving put-downs. I thought of times I had been in similar situations. The wealth of people skills that had been important and available to me on Earth was now vividly apparent in the spiritual realm where I was shown truth.

I became aware of some of the challenges of women involved in arguments because their mates wanted only their own opinion or decision to be accepted as the final word, with no discussion or allowance for expression of a differing viewpoint, opinion, or expansion on their idea. This need caused some women to feel frustrated and to develop pent-up feelings of anger. Other women unleashed harsh words which fueled heated arguments.

Yet I knew relationships on Earth could be revitalized if people kept in mind the answer after asking themselves: "How important will this argument be in one hundred years? Even in one hundred days?"

Another couple I saw arguing was, again, one spouse trying to change the other's opinion. I could see that their argument was a waste of time. The more the man bickered and badgered and belittled his wife, the stronger she came back at him with her opinions and accusations. I could feel what she was feeling and I understood why she believed the way she did.

The wife was at a different level of growth than her husband. She thought she was absolutely justified in her beliefs. He, on the other hand, was coming from his level of growth and beliefs. He was feeling greatly frustrated and he could not comprehend why his wife couldn't see his point of view. Childishly, neither person would step back and allow the other to have a different opinion. They didn't even try to see the situation from the other person's viewpoint and neither would let go of their own opinions.

A Coping Technique—Let It Go

I learned an important concept: *Let it go.* I realized there was so much energy wasted in trying to prove oneself right. Arguing over ideas and opinions can ruin relationships. As each person uses words that hurt, it is as if he or she is lighting the fires of anger in the other. Harsh words only add to the other person's anger and they feel more inflamed—it is like trying to put out a fire by throwing on gasoline. Leaving opinions unchallenged can be much wiser.

Watching these couples argue while feeling their real emotions gave me new understandings, patience, and acceptance of others' opinions. It helped me realize how much time I had wasted in contentions and arguments. I became aware that being *unwilling* to see another's viewpoint or not taking time to communicate so *another understands properly* always damages relationships.

The importance and wisdom of listening with an understanding heart and communicating without criticizing and putting others down was impressed upon my mind as I understood the far-reaching consequences and effects of words.

Loving Words Are a Healing Balm

More knowledge came into my mind and I became aware of many benefits of loving unconditionally—especially the importance of *expressing loving words*. I knew that people need to feel loved and to be **told they are loved**. Sincere loving words can be a healing balm to the soul of someone who is hurting.

Thoughts came to my mind of some of the many times in my life when I had yearned to feel loved. I knew that I was not alone. Usually women, even more than men, long to hear those precious words, "I love you."

I wondered why it was so difficult for most men to understand women's feelings; why it was usually difficult for them to express loving words. With that thought, it was as though I could see through a man's eyes and feel with a man's heart. I suddenly knew how different men's perspectives are from women's and that women can be extremely difficult for them to understand. With this new awareness, I realized how difficult it is for most men to express their feelings and emotions, and that generally, it is easier and more natural for women to talk about what bothers them.

Men usually don't know what a woman means when she says she doesn't *feel* loved, or when she wants to discuss all the things that upset her. Men usually believe they are *showing* love by working hard for their families, and they often think that loving words are unnecessary. Usually the man does not know how to respond and may withdraw— the opposite response the woman wants.

I realized that some of this lack came from the example of parents who did not express their feelings—traditions handed down from generation to generation. Also, the people were created with definite differences in temperaments and emotions for many good reasons. However, I knew that situations and people could change as they react and adapt to each other's differences.

Arguments Have No "Victor"

From these scenes I viewed on the Other Side, I became aware that quarreling over differences does not lead to solutions, and arguments are never actually "won." If a "victory" hurts another there is no real victory. The couples I saw arguing did not have clear goals; arguing had become a habit and was destructive to the self-esteem of those involved—especially to the tender feelings of children.

The people in these arguments did not realize that they displayed their own faults when they raised their voices for emphasis, shouted, and used profanity to make an impression. It was observable that they were without adequate words in their vocabulary and that they were trying to sound smarter, more "right," speaking in this manner. Being unwilling or unable to communicate effectively, they shouted put-downs.

At times they laughed at others or became angry or labeled them "stupid" for not agreeing with their opinions or for not following their instructions. They did not see that the failing was their own—they were not communicating adequately.

Watching these couples locked in useless arguing and knowing the feelings of each partner, I became aware that people skills—especially communication skills—are a vital part of the mortal experience. Whether or not we choose to learn them will

CHAPTER 26

How to Gain Mercy—Not Justice!

In my life review, I saw times where I had been offended or hurt by someone and also times when I had been the one causing an offense. I watched the way I acted or reacted. I experienced the same thoughts and felt the feelings I had at those moments, and I knew the thoughts and experienced the feelings of other individuals involved. This gave me a new profound awakening and awareness of my senses, and my consciousness was filled with understanding of our motivations. At the time I had misjudged others because I did not know *their* viewpoints. I regretted making a big issue of seeking justice. I had wanted those who seemed to deliberately hurt others, to "pay" for their behavior.

I was critical and would get upset when people who appeared cruel or unfair to others would prosper from their ruthlessness. I thought that they did not have many trials or tribulations, but led happy lives. In contrast, I wondered why many humble, kind people seemed to trudge through life having to bear numerous hardships and trials.

Things Are Infinitely Fair on the Other Side

When my awareness was expanded to view situations in their proper eternal perspective, *I knew that after someone had lived his or her life and gone to the Other Side, they would face their actions, and no one would get ahead unfairly.* Good deeds, small and large, would be rewarded and bad ones would reap punishment.

Gathering Good Deeds for Other-Side Enjoyment

I realized that Earth time had been my time for gathering kind thoughts, deeds, and actions for enjoyment on the Other Side. I wish I could adequately describe the feelings I felt, the sorrow I experienced to have criticized or misjudged another of God's children in any way during my journey through life. In instances where I'd hurt another's feelings, I felt deep remorse.

Also, I knew that if someone hurts another and seems to get away with it, as if robbing justice while alive on Earth, there was no need wishing revenge on them. If someone does not seem to have a conscience on Earth, it does not mean that they do not have one; they do and it will pain them with an agony later. They are really hurting themselves.

As We Judge, So Shall We Be Judged

However, instead of being relieved or grateful that others would someday have to pay for their behavior, I felt sorrow for them as I realized that they were losing their other-side rewards and bringing punishment on themselves. With my new and increased understanding of eternal rewards and eternal punishments, I no longer wanted revenge or retaliation against anyone for anything. I knew that it was a Great Universal Truth that what we give out comes back to us. As we judge others we will be judged. As we sow, so shall we reap.

Forgive to Be Forgiven

I knew that if I wanted to receive mercy, I needed to give mercy while I was alive. I wanted to be able to forgive anyone and everyone who had offended me. I discovered that it was literally true that we earn what we receive on the Other Side by the choices we make while on the Earth. As I experienced my life review and understood things in their proper perspective, I saw that each time I had wished justice on another I was determining the way I would judge myself.

Glorious Feelings Come from Being Kind

Then the thought forcefully came to my mind that if what I give out is truly what I get back, I didn't want justice, I wanted mercy! I knew that if I wanted to receive mercy, I would had to have given mercy while I was alive. I wanted to return to Earth life and be merciful to others. Also, I knew that if I had intentionally offended one of God's children, it was an offense to God.

I knew for myself what I had done or not done on Earth and glorious feelings of joy accompanied the good I had done, especially for those who seemed to deserve it least.

God Loves All Creatures

More knowledge came to my mind with a sharp awareness of truth about the importance of being kind and merciful not only to people, but to all of God's creatures: animals, birds, reptiles, etc. God's love extends to His creatures in all their wondrous variety and so should ours. I knew that they were placed on Earth for wise purposes and that they are not to be intentionally mistreated.

All of the knowledge I had been shown added to my understanding of the importance of the time on Earth and the joy I could have reaped if I had spent more of my time giving mercy rather than seeking justice. *The heavenly rewards that can be earned are worth the effort!*

This truth touched my soul and gave great meaning to the Biblical teaching, "But glory, honour, and peace, to every man that worketh good…" (Romans 2:10)

CHAPTER 27

A Source of Joy Beyond Comprehension

Abruptly, I was again aware of the question from the Being of Light. As He repeated it to me, it pierced my consciousness. He asked, "What did you do with what you had in life?" This question had nothing to do with the blessings *other* people received in their lives, or what others had done with *their* circumstances in life. Rather, I absolutely knew again that I was not competing against anyone else's good works; there was no one else to blame for my omissions. He was asking me only what I did with what I *did* have. My sins of omission became very obvious to me—there were things I did *not* do that I should have done with what I was given, such as being more charitable, patient, and helpful to others.

My chance at mortal life's opportunities to grow mentally and spiritually was finished. I wanted to run, to hide—anything to not have to face the reality that I'd not done what I could have during my Earth life. But I knew that my own thoughts and actions had earned what I was experiencing.

Unconditional Love—a Source of Peace

Then, I thought of some of the little good deeds I had done for others that only they and I knew, such as when I took time to cheer and visit someone who needed encouragement, especially when it was not convenient. These were things that I thought to be insignificant at the time.

However, in the Spiritual realm, I was benefitting from small acts of kindness in a much larger way. The joy I received from my little kind deeds was magnified and I realized that God was pleased when one of His children helps another one. Precious feelings of joy flooded over me and I knew that *all* compassionate acts of charity and kindness, *even small ones*, reap joy and great rewards. Also, I understood the importance of true, unconditional love for others. Every word or action motivated by love, not because someone did something for me first, brought peace to my soul.

I knew God had set the example for us by loving every one of us unconditionally. As I thought of this, my being was infused again with total love from the God of Love and Light. I felt love radiate from Him all through and around me. God's love was so magnificent that it vastly expanded my feelings of love and empathy for others. I marveled that I could feel that deeply, that *anyone* could feel that much love.

As more knowledge expanded my consciousness, it became clear that a higher way of living could be accomplished on Earth. It required constant choices to avoid condemning, gossiping, criticizing, and judging others.

Even though it would be a continual day-to-day challenge for most everyone, I knew there would be more lasting happiness while living on Earth for those who strive to avoid judging others. Family traditions and personal traits of being loving and forgiving could be handed down to posterity by example and all could reap eternal rewards.

Accepting Differences Brings Freedom

I became aware that appreciating others and their differences promotes creativity and diversity and enjoyment. It became clear there are differences in people's likes and their actions according to their age, experience, and family influence. I knew it would be sad if we all had the same likes and dislikes; things would look dull if everyone wanted the same color and kind of cars, houses, or clothes. Suddenly I knew that diversity makes the world an interesting and colorful place.

Learning from Choices

Then I knew that accepting people at their own level of growth and patiently letting them learn from their choices can bring peace and joy beyond description. Acceptance would bring a form of freedom—freedom from pettiness, from prejudice, from judging and being judged. The freedom I felt was wonderful as I understood that each person has different interests and goals and was to be permitted to learn from the results of their choices.

More knowledge came to my mind that there are immeasurable benefits for not judging people's actions, looks, or differences. I understood that when people felt accepted and were permitted to make their free-will choices, they could more easily grow to their personal potential.

At this point, I was understanding things from the perspective of eternal growth, viewing all phases of a situation, all sides, along with the feelings of those involved. I could see the results, the repercussions of my wrongful decisions or indecisions.

The Truth and Beauty of the Scriptures

My thoughts turned to the scriptures and I was impressed with their truthfulness, beauty, and the rewards to be gained by learning and striving to live God's teachings. I was amazed to realize how literally true and wise the scriptures are. I knew that just reading their words could never do them justice, but by pondering them also, more of their meaning could be recognized.

We Cannot Fool God or Ourselves

My every action or reaction, I found, went out in time like unending circles that somehow came back to me. Anything I did or did not do for anyone else had an effect that came back to me. I could no more fool God into thinking I had done my best with my time on Earth than I could fool myself.

I Wanted to Shout from the Housetops

Wanting to return to my body on Earth to apply what I had learned, I wanted desperately to be able to speak. I felt that if I were given the chance to tell others, I would shout from the rooftops what I had learned: *the importance of being forgiving and the countless blessings that can be reaped by being kind, merciful, and by loving unconditionally.*

Still, I believed my plea was in vain. I had made my choice. The saddest experience I ever had was to recognize all the things I could *no longer do* and to know that I could not make any corrections to my choices. I was racked with torment as I realized that I could no longer even attempt to repent and do better in life.

Forgiving for My Sake

On Earth, I had taken classes that taught a *false* process for getting over offenses: First, tell those involved how much they had hurt me. Second, talk it out. Third, receive an apology from the offender(s) and fourth, let it go. Mistakenly, however, I was told I was to receive an apology from the offender before I moved on.

When my knowledge was expanded, to my surprise I discovered I was not to tell someone how I felt about them and then forgive them. I was to forgive others unconditionally and treat others as I would want to be treated, not just for their sake, but for *mine*, because of how I would feel about myself and my actions. Forgiving, forgetting, and letting go of grudges brings benefits for all concerned, whether offenders apologize and ask for forgiveness or not.

Knowing that the sooner I rid myself of feeling offended, the better off I would be. I saw that I could have gained peace of mind in the mortal world and had more peace in the Spiritual realm if I'd done this. I knew that anger at *anyone* hurt me mentally, physically, and especially spiritually.

Even though there was a different sense of "time" on the Other Side, I realized I had learned a lot and had seen many scenes since my transition from Earth life to the Spirit World. At that time, I thought that I might be caught endlessly in this awful state where I was filled with feelings of remorse.

Forgive before It's Too Late

Suddenly, I felt myself moving through a space of dense blackness and through the midst of miserable souls who had died while still holding onto angry, bitter grudges toward others. They carried their dark, angry feelings with them in the Spirit realm, and they could not let go of them. Wanting to escape the angry feelings, I found myself floating away from the darkness and through space. Coming down through a beam of light, I found myself looking into a room in a hospital. I saw an older man lying in a hospital bed blankly staring toward the end of his bed and upward toward the ceiling.

98

I wondered if he could see me looking down on him, but then I knew he could not. Drifting into and out of consciousness, he was too weak to move or communicate with the man and woman standing at the side of his bed. By mental communication, I knew that the woman about his same age was his wife, and the younger man was his son.

Also I realized that the father had been very angry with his son and had not spoken to him for years, except with extremely harsh words. The mother and son felt that his bad feelings had added to the deterioration of the father's health. The son had avoided further contact; each believed the other should apologize. Now, with the father's impending death, there was great sadness displayed on the faces and in the words of the mother and son. The son had tears rolling down his cheeks and his voice broke as he said, "Dad, I'm so sorry for hurting you. Please forgive me; I love you. Please forgive me, Dad." He repeated the words many times, as he cried and asked for forgiveness.

I understood the son's sorrow. He knew it was too late; his father was dying and could not respond. But the young man continued trying to make himself heard and to apologize. It was easy to observe that the young man felt tremendous guilt knowing he had waited too long to speak the precious words his father wanted to hear but that he could not previously bring himself to say, "I am sorry. I love you."

The son turned toward his mother and tearfully said, "Mom, I am so sorry for not apologizing to Dad before. I know I have hurt us all. I am sorry I wasn't there when Dad needed me." He turned back to his father and continued crying and apologizing but still with no response from the father.

The mother lowered her head as she softly cried, too. I understood her pained emotions; she felt torn between her son and husband, and she had lost the enjoyment of them both over this family feud. Her sadness was intensified now, for the two of them and for herself.

Watching them, I wondered how long this young man would feel these terrible feelings of remorse. I did not receive an answer, but I recognized many of my own foolish feelings when I had been involved in futile arguments and waited for another person to apologize. I now recognized the value of putting a relationship ahead of receiving words of apology.

"Time" Is Too Limited to Hold Grudges

Many people, I now knew, feel offended and wait for the other to take the first step in the forgiving process—to call and say they are sorry. They wait to hear those most priceless words, "I love you." But when they are close to death they have painful feelings of wanting to be able to communicate their love. I knew that when they were finally facing death, they no longer wanted to express anger, but rather, they wanted to ask for forgiveness, express love, and feel the other's love in return.

No one on Earth knows for sure when their time may unexpectedly run out, when it will be too late to communicate their love. I thought of my own circumstances and I knew that time is too limited to waste holding grudges, being angry, and withholding love.

Forgiveness Brings Glorious Freedom

We take our feelings with us when we die. Those who are patient with others, who are able to forgive when feeling offended and let go of anger on Earth, experience great feelings of glorious freedom and inner peace on the Other Side. They reap joy beyond comprehension.

When my understanding was opened, I sincerely sorrowed for those who hold grudges, intentionally hurt another's feelings, or try to take advantage of others. They would not do or say hurtful things if they realized the seemingly unending ripples of repercussions from regrettable actions. Decisions to hurt others result in lost opportunities for reaping joy and eternal peace of mind.

CHAPTER 28

The Truth That Brings Self-Worth and Personal Power

Throughout my life I had struggled to feel confident. I had not been happy with my weight or my appearance. Most of my life I felt I was too heavy or too old or too ill. When I looked in the mirror, my attention focused on my physical imperfections.

On the Other Side, I gained an entirely different impression of my body. When I watched my life review, it became clear what a valuable gift my body was and how necessary it was to accomplish what I desired to do during Earth life. I didn't need to be unhappy because I did not look a certain way or was not the same size as someone else. The important thing was that I *had* a body. It had been dependent on how I treated it; if I had kept it healthy it could have served me well rather than hindered my progress during my life's journey.

In the spiritual realm, I realized how my own poor health habits (such as not eating properly, not getting enough rest or exercise, or pushing myself to the point of exhaustion) had impacted my health and body.

Too late, I learned that my body was precious and vitally important for many reasons and that without it I could not even pick up a piece of paper. My Earthly body had many limitations, many ailments, and had caused me much pain, but I had not realized it gave me freedom as well—the freedom to act, to do the things I chose to do, and to participate in Earthly experiences.

Unfinished Business

I anguished about important things I wanted to return to Earth to do or finish that I could only accomplish with a body. While I was alive on Earth I had been unhappy about what I could not do that I had believed my body would not let me do. I had more patience for someone else's physical limitations than my own.

On the Other Side, I saw the importance of prioritizing time and tasks in order to accomplish more and still have energy left for the next day. While I was alive on Earth, I did not like wasting time and it seemed nonproductive to rest when there was so much to be done. If I had only realized the truth about health, taking care of the body, and the wise use of time, including resting when needed, I could have enjoyed my journey through life with better health.

I became aware that there is an *energy-force reserve* available to draw from during life on Earth. When I made withdrawals from the reservoir of energy I needed to put life-giving things back into it by eating the right foods, maintaining a good mental attitude, taking care of relationships by doing things for others. These were important keys to keep the body's energy reserves filled and make possible Earthly enjoyment and heavenly rewards.

Feeling Chained to Circumstances

During my Earth life, I had taken self-improvement classes, but I still needed more confidence. There were times I believed my timid feelings and attitudes helplessly chained me to my circumstances. As I relived these feelings, suddenly a scene was presented to my view that was symbolic of what I had thought about and how I had felt. I saw myself lying on a bright, sandy beach flat on my back. Heavy chains across my limbs bound me tightly and held me firmly against the hot sand. Lifting my head, I could see that the oppressive chains were too strong for me to escape.

As I examined them, I realized and understood what they really were: my own feelings of inadequacy. They were all the put-downs from other people, my own negative self-talk, my painful feelings of incompetence, and perceived lack of abilities.

The Freedom of Truth

The chains held me so that I was hardly able to move. I wondered how I had been able to function in my life with such strong chains binding me. The situation seemed hopeless, and I felt completely unable to help myself.

Just when I was about to give in to complete despair, I felt an infusion of love from God. My mind opened to the knowledge of my true nature; I was not just another life form, *I was a child of God.*

True Empowerment Comes from God

My thoughts centered on that incredible Being of Love and Light who stood by my side. Feelings of empowerment, self-worth, confidence, and the unconquerable courage to be myself immediately filled my being. My inferiority complex was gone. All negative thoughts suddenly disappeared, replaced with my new awareness of reality.

The limits I had put on myself came to mind, and I knew that in Earth life I did not need to be chained down with feelings of inadequacy. My self-worth was not dependent on other people. I was important to God, was one of His creations, and I knew He loved me. I realized that God is no respecter of fame or fortune. *Everyone is important to Him—and to themselves.*

This view and understanding filled me with gratitude and a feeling of being loved. Then I sensed a feeling of freedom. In that state of mind I moved my arm; I saw that it came up freely. Amazed, I turned to look at my other arm; it was free also. The chains I had thought were so strong were actually insubstantial and powerless to hold me. Kicking my legs, I found them free as well, and now I was completely free!

Standing, I turned and looked back at the sand where I had lain so hopelessly bound just a few moments before. The chains of self-doubt had melted; they were gone. How could this be? The chains that had hampered me all my life had lacked substance and truth. No one had unlocked them, no one pulled them away from me, yet they now had no power over me. Only one thing made the difference between freedom and captivity: knowledge of my importance to God and to myself.

Dispelling False Beliefs Brings Personal Power

No person had unlocked my chains because no other person had the power to do so. The only power they had ever had was the power of my belief in them. They had seemed and felt so real, but they were *not* real—they were of my own making. They were a hoax, a trick I had played

103

on myself. But no mental chains were strong enough to bind me when I realized that I was a child of God and had great personal power.

Although I didn't realize it, I always had the power to stand and walk away from my chains of self-doubt and low self-esteem. I had within me the power to dispel the dark untruths I had believed about myself throughout my life. The knowledge of my true nature turned on the light in my inner self and illuminated my path to freedom.

When I thought back on the many books I had read and courses I had taken that I had thought were fantastic, now they all seemed trivial. All the books and courses in the world were nothing when compared with the knowledge and confidence I gained when I actually realized I *was a child of God*.

Programming the Computer of the Mind

While on the Other Side, I learned that the mind was like a powerful computer that needed to be constantly cared for with proper input. Otherwise, the product it produced would be of poor quality—and that product is *who* we are.

Vividly I realized how important it was to avoid self-disparaging thoughts that would produce unwanted results. Such thoughts when allowed to stay in my mind had formed the chains that pulled me down and hindered my growth.

I realized that my mind was powerful, but it was also my servant, a part of my Earthly body given me to use wisely; I was in charge. I could have taken command of my thinking and my attitudes. I could have worked at keeping my mind on things I wanted instead of on things I worried about. On Earth, I could have re-programmed my thinking—because I was a child of God.

Self-worth and personal power, I learned, are **not** a result of looking or acting a certain way or achieving a certain amount. They come from knowing and remembering the truth: *I am a child of God.*

CHAPTER 29

Scenes of Premortality

Suddenly, the scenes in my life review were gone and scenes of my premortal life came into view. I was aware that I was part of a large group of enthusiastic supporters of the planned Earth life. Immediately I knew I was not born on Earth simply by chance. There were reasons—eternal purposes for everything. I knew about the Earth's creation and had a great love for it.

Everything was designed to fit together and function in harmony, and I observed that each part has a reason for being; each part supports all other parts by its existence— even insects. Things I had taken for granted or thought of as insignificant now had new importance. All things, I now knew, are significant and necessary to help the Earth be whole and complete.

For example, water—an everyday substance—is important in every aspect of life on Earth. Next, I knew the importance of trees that purify the air, filtering it and creating oxygen. I was never fond of trees and vegetation before. My favorite landscaping would have been almost exclusively rocks.

That changed when I knew how important trees are and how dependent everything is on everything else. Trees, vegetation, and seeds took on a new significance for me. How gloriously everything functioned; how marvelously it was created! I had a new respect and appreciation for all of God's creations. The love I had for Earth was tremendous. It was incredibly important to me as I realized the significance of it in the plan and miracle of creation.

In the premortal world, I saw that it was Earth life that would allow me the opportunity to have a mortal body and mortal experiences. My understanding increased as I realized why our memories of premortal life have to be hidden with an Earthly veil of forgetfulness: *so that we can **gain wisdom**—learn, develop mentally and spiritually, find joy through obedience, and become more loving, charitable, and forgiving.* Also, I realized that I could not have functioned properly on Earth if I had remembered the joy of being engulfed in Godly love. The longing would have been so great to be back in His presence that I could not have withstood the pain.

I Chose to Come to Earth

When I was on the Other Side, I wondered about life before birth, and whether I had wanted to be born or had any choice about it. My question was answered profoundly in these quick glimpses of premortality. I distinctly remembered with a burst of happiness some of the excitement I had felt about coming to Earth. I knew I was not alone in this excitement; all of us were eager to participate in this plan. We were not *lukewarm* about this; we were exuberant. With this realization and refreshing of my memory, I felt repentant for having wondered whether I had wanted to be born—the answer was so obviously yes.

Each of Us Has a Purpose

My remembrance of the premortal world while on the Other Side reawakened my feelings and knowledge about the wonders connected to being born, having a body, and being part of this eternal plan. With a bright awareness, I recalled that I wanted to help make the Earth a better place for those who would come after me and be part of the whole.

My birth on Earth was for a purpose which I accepted and wanted to accomplish. I wanted to be part of the group who were creating benefits for others in the world. I knew that each choice made on Earth can have far-reaching effects. Every person and every choice matters more than we can realize at the time.

I was amazed at what I was shown and what I learned from glimpses of premortal life, scenes of the spirit world, and revelations of knowledge that were impressed upon my consciousness. The events in premortality and Earth life only fit together when viewed from life on the Other Side.

The additional knowledge was given to me that the Earth is for all of God's children, and the responsibility for it belongs to all of us. However, there are many who come to Earth who do not realize or care about its importance. Knowing that the Earth was being fouled by some for whom it was created, whose lives depended on it, caused me to feel great sadness.

Every Person and Every Creature Matters to God

It was painful to observe those who mistreat other people under their care, including helpless children and the elderly. Their pain when confronted with their own actions will be worse than that which they inflicted.

Thoughts came to my mind of those who regrettably discount the intelligence, emotions, and feelings of pain of animals—and any creatures on Earth—sometimes because they didn't care and sometimes because they did not realize the eternal nature of God's creations. I knew that many people on Earth greatly underestimate how much God cares about His animals and other creatures and how people treat them. It was sad that many who had high possibilities fell short of their potential in their treatment of their families, others, and defenseless creatures.

It was exciting to learn of the tremendous joy awaiting those who accept their challenges and make it through them while striving to keep God's commandments—they then reap their earned rewards. I had an overwhelming desire to be among the group on Earth who serve Him and do His will.

However, many of my own free-will choices while I was alive on Earth had brought me feelings of remorse instead.

CHAPTER 30

Eternal Perspectives

My life review continued and my attention focused on scenes with my mother. I became aware of thoughts I'd had on Earth such as, "Why didn't I have someone else as my mother or my father?" I heard my thoughts: "My life would have been so much better if I had had different parents. I could have accomplished so much more." It was as though those thoughts were visible around me. I tried to escape from them, but I could not.

Just as suddenly, other things were in my view and I knew that I had chosen my mother although I wasn't told this was the case for everyone else. I had *wanted* to be her daughter, not for the things she could do for me on Earth, but for what I could do for her. She needed me! She was a special, precious person who needed my help to make it through her journey of Earth life. In her own way, she was hurting as much as I had been.

I Was Wrong about Being Right

Our lives together had been filled with contention and arguments over what was truth and who was right. We had often used words that hurt each other and our relationship had been extremely frustrating for both of us. It seemed we were always angry with each other.

For years I had longed to hear her tell me she loved me and that she was sorry about my unhappy childhood. I wanted her to accept me but I felt I could never please her. We argued over big things and little things. A poem came to mind that I had written when I was a teenager expressing my mistaken feelings about being right. The poem reads:

Oh Mother dear, I sadly fear
that until we die
we will continue to try
to argue and fight
to prove who is right
although we both know, I am.

108

Erroneously, I had believed that finding out who was "right" would cure almost any situation. I had falsely believed that a vigorous pursuit of justice in all things was essential, as if it would automatically stop wrongful actions as soon as "truth" was discovered. The stark reality of how false this notion was became clear to me. I discovered how wrong I was to quarrel about being right and saw that everyone believes, or likes to think they're right.

Who was right or wrong, whether she was sorry or not, or whether she told me she loved me was no longer a concern. Oh, how my feelings for my mother and my understanding of her changed. No longer did I feel compelled to have her say or do something to show she loved me. I knew of her love for me. I *felt* her feelings as though I had been her.

My Mother Needed Me

My awareness exploded with the information and reality of how much my mother needed me. My love for her blossomed and I realized her heartaches and life's trials. I missed her in this spiritual sphere and I wanted to help her and talk to her; I was saddened and frustrated that I could not. As I realized this, my feelings of remorse intensified. I had let us both down. Also, I knew that she had a difficult time telling me she loved me and she needed me to tell her I loved her.

The foolishness and futility of bickering and fighting with anyone was impressed upon me. I was very sorry for wasting irreplaceable time senselessly arguing about happenings, situations, opinions, and who was right. My sorrow was extreme for every harsh or sharp word I had ever spoken to anyone, especially family members. If you want to strengthen the relationship, it's far more important to help others save face than trying prove them wrong.

We Learn from Each Other

Also, I saw that people watch and learn from each other and repeat each other's actions and mistakes. It became clear to me how everyone's *actions* influence the basic lives of countless others

Quickly, new scenes came to my view containing additional, important messages for me. I saw a mother teaching her daughter to clean a floor thoroughly. Her voice was sweet as she approvingly said, "The floor looks nice and clean, but that corner could look better and needs to be redone." The mother's words conveyed her love and acceptance and did not make the girl feel rejected but motivated her to improve her skills. I understood that the mother's object was not only to get the floor clean, but to instill confidence in her child and to teach her good work habits for life.

Again, the scene before me changed swiftly and I saw another mother belittling her child for not doing the chores according to *her* standards. The mother grabbed the cleaning cloth from her daughter and said in a sharp tone of voice, "Why do I have to do everything myself? You are so clumsy, you can't do anything right." Then she did the task herself. I saw the young child cringe as she developed habitual feelings of inferiority and depression that would lead her toward giving up.

I became aware that the ultimate goal in teaching children is to help them learn and mature so that they can succeed without being supervised. They need a safe family environment in order to gain wisdom, confidence, and the experience of doing things on their own. They need an *inner* desire to do things correctly, not because they are being watched or because someone makes them perform their tasks to an acceptable standard.

Entrusted to My Care

This was an enlightening revelation for me. I wanted to cry out to my children—to apologize for the times I was impatient with them as they went through their learning experiences during childhood. Then I also knew that my children were actually *God's* children entrusted to my care. From this perspective, I understood that the problems that came up as I was raising them were really opportunities for us to learn some of life's valuable lessons, such as the connection between choices and consequences.

I had always loved my children, but now I had gained a vivid new understanding of how extremely important and precious they were. Also, I missed them in this sphere and I longed to be able to talk to them. I wanted to tell them about things they could do on Earth that would help them prepare for their journey to the Other Side.

Teaching Opportunities Are Fleeting

Rapidly, scenes from priceless child-rearing years passed for my review. The swift passage of the time I had with my children brought the distinct realization that my best opportunities for teaching them were gone—in fact *all* opportunities to be with them or to teach them on Earth were *gone*.

When I was alive on Earth, I had seen a wall plaque with a saying on it, "Life was what happened while I was busy with other plans." I was struck in this spiritual realm with the actuality of that statement. Before I realized it, those brief childhood times while my children's questioning minds were so open and accepting of ideas had passed, never to be recaptured.

I looked back over the years when my children were small with their minds absorbing my philosophies and attitudes as they matured. I heard words I had said many times as they were growing up, and winced: "Who's at fault? Tell the truth—what happened here? We have to be fair about this. You are wrong."

Those parenting phrases seemed normal; they were ones I often heard in my own childhood and so repeated as a parent. I wanted to raise my children to seek fairness and justice. That was how I had been raised and how my mother had been raised.

The scenes I viewed while I was on the Other Side revealed to me the error of seeking "truth" and "fairness" over teaching forgiveness and tolerance. Being right or establishing fault faded into insignificance compared to being concerned about feelings, building character, and developing self-esteem while children are young and most open to training.

Words Can Hurt

As quickly as my mind comprehended these scenes, my vision expanded to the view of many little children. I felt the feelings of these small children as they took harsh verbal attacks from parents locked into patterns of false child-rearing notions that went back several generations (including put-downs and words that battered self-images, words that could hurt like a blow from a fist).

I saw parents yelling at their children, who in frustration and anger falsely believed they were reacting normally to their situations. The children

111

absorbed like little sponges the tone of their parent's voices and the tensions around them. Like little tape recorders, they were recording in their minds the words they heard their parents use.

Mental Tape Recorders

Then I saw those same children as adults with their children. It was as though someone hit the playback button on their mental tape recorders. They were using their parents' impatient and ineffective responses word for word. They were parenting the way they had been taught, following their parents' unsuccessful example.

My children came into my view and I knew how precious and important they were as part of my life. Each child had been like a jewel I was given on Earth to care for, lovingly polish, and help develop its special radiance. I loved them very much and wanted to communicate with them. My love and concern for them was infinitely more than it was while I was with them in Earth life. I had no idea the "spiritual sphere" was this way. I wanted to go back to Earth to warn them not to repeat the mistakes I had made.

Suddenly my feelings of remorse in regard to my lack of parenting skills ceased. Wait! I thought defensively, I had not been given an "owner's manual" when I had my first child, nor had my mother. I was doing the best I knew how, and so had my mother and her parents. We believed we were doing right at the time. In reality, we were functioning at our own level of growth, just as everyone does.

Excuses Melt in the Bright Light of Truth

I also realized that people can break free of undesirable teachings and habits, including undesired family traditions. It is not easy, yet it can be done with the help of the Creator through the power of prayer and a person's own self-determination. My excuses continued to melt in the bright light of truth.

The perspectives I gained about all the members of my family cast a new light of understanding on the importance of every pattern handed down from one generation to another. I wanted to change many of the ones that were being handed down to my posterity—but now I could not.

CHAPTER 31

Mingling with Angels

As soon as I grasped the meaning of these scenes, I found myself quickly traveling through time and space through a star-filled blackness. Suddenly, I stopped. I clearly saw parenting patterns being passed downward from my children, to theirs, and onward. Also, I saw generations of people from many lands and cultures continuing with family experiences and traditions, good or bad.

The Being of Love and Light was just a short distance from me and was showing me the spirits of many people whom I somehow knew were several generations of *my* posterity.

Then I saw a beautiful young woman with lovely dark hair and beautiful blue eyes. I couldn't stop staring at her; I felt drawn to her. As our eyes met, she smiled and held out her arms toward me. But she paused and with her arms still outstretched she said, "I've waited so long." Putting her arms down, she then turned and was gone. I knew that one day she would be born to one of my descendants.

In 1983, while I was on the Other Side in the Spirit World, I was among many adult spirits and mingling with angels. They were all around me and as I passed through their midst I had a deep understanding that many of them would be my posterity on Earth.

Family Is More Important than Success

I was struck with the knowledge of how important the family and home life are—more important than anything else. Any other success is temporary. I knew that gaining all the success the world has to offer is meaningless compared to the family.

Even though we are often away from our families because of reasons we cannot control, I knew that we can all make a greater effort to spend quality time together. If parents made a greater effort to set a better example for their children by being more empathetic, loving, and nurturing, it would have a profound effect on their children for many generations to come. With this awareness, as I looked at all these precious ones, I knew now that all actions, large and small, good or bad, can have eternal consequences.

As soon as I had that thought, I thought of children playing games and heard the soft "Ping, Ping, Ping" when they had scored points as they played the same game over and over again. Their concentration is intense. I had a burning feeling that there are other things they need to do and learn, things that would help them in their mortal development.

Spending so much time playing unproductive games, watching mindless television, or randomly surfing the web creates a void in their development. Instead, they should be learning the great lessons of life, things that they can pass on to others. They waited a long time for the opportunity to have mortal bodies and their precious time is too often squandered in front of a screen that the parents purchased for them and taught them how to use. I wanted to return to Earth life to share this new understanding with parents and young people alike.

Looking at the posterity of generations all around me, I sadly realized that parents' lack of child-rearing skills would contribute to some of the unhappiness they would have when they went to Earth. Challenges resulting from the inadequacy of parents would ricochet through time. I knew of some of the trials they would go through in their lives; troubles caused by knowledge they lacked because their parents didn't teach their children, and they, in turn, didn't teach theirs, and so on.

There were things they would not learn on Earth which would have greatly benefitted them. I saw how the lack of knowledge of certain important life lessons could be traced back from one generation to the preceding generation, all the way back, in some cases, to early ancestors. During my Earth life, I had never thought of these things, but in the spirit world, they were apparent.

My anguish intensified as I understood the far-reaching effects of not helping our children and grandchildren learn more worthwhile things. When they miss out on these precious growing experiences they lose out on eternal rewards that they may have otherwise gained as they taught their children and grandchildren, and as they, in turn, taught their children and grandchildren and so on.

Gaining Wisdom, a Grand Key to Happiness

I saw that gaining wisdom and overcoming problems are some of the grand keys God gives us to unlock our own happiness and the growth and happiness of our posterity and those around us. I saw how loving parenting skills would help all concerned. Also, I realized the importance of believing that situations and relationships can improve and then working to better things rather than being quick to judge and give up on a family member.

As I mingled with angels and those whom I knew were to be my posterity, my understanding was opened and I knew that these parenting skills were some of the important lessons that were to be learned in the school of life.

CHAPTER 32

Fads and Fashions—Whirling through Time & Space

Suddenly, I was again whirling through time and space. My view opened to new scenes; I saw the history of the world unfold on a huge panoramic screen. Life seemed like a puzzle with pieces falling into place. It was so exhilarating! I thought of how people on Earth think programs on TV or in movies are exciting, but they pale when compared to our own fascinating world's history.

I had heard a lot of negative things about the world and its history, but just as in my own day, in years past much good had gone unnoticed. It probably always would until everything is known on the Other Side.

I saw that fashions and standards of beauty changed over the years. My attention focused on a scene where I saw a fairly large, portly woman who was considered a true beauty in her time. She was posing semi-nude for a painting, and I realized that everyone could someday view not only the painting, but her posing for it.

Instantly, I knew she felt proud to be posing for this painting but there would come a time when she would regret it. At this moment, however, she was proud of herself, her beauty, and her roly-poly figure. I chuckled when I thought of all the poor thin women of her day who envied her full figure. They disliked their looks and felt lacking in feminine beauty because their bodies did not match their time-period's standard of loveliness when it was fashionable to be plump.

Beauty Standards Are Passing Fads

The beauty standard in my time was almost an exact opposite. I learned that the *fat* or *thin* question was a *passing fad* that passed with time and was not important in heaven. With a stark realization, I knew that while on Earth we may be teased or belittled if our size or looks do not match the

116

current standard of beauty. However, the standards by which we are judged on Earth change often and are not of lasting significance.

I knew that a healthy body at an ideal weight for each person's frame (not thin) would become fashionable. I was surprised to learn this about weight; it was such a big issue during my lifetime. I was surprised to learn that being overweight did not reap ridicule on the Other Side as it does on Earth. However, there is obvious wisdom in eating right.

Heavenly Treasures Don't Go Out of Style

"People and family are more important than things"

Glimpses of men and women were shown me who desired to be in style and in vogue with fashions that changed with the whims and fads of their time. I knew that they sacrificed important things in their lives for fancy clothes, jewelry, and other material things, to stay at the height of whatever was considered the "in thing" at the time. It seemed silly to me from my Other Side viewpoint, and I learned how important it was to keep a balance. Priorities needed to be grounded by an eternal perspective of heavenly treasures that did not wear out or go out of style.

As the years passed and styles changed, I saw that apparel which had been so important lost its appeal as the newest or latest fashion was desired instead. After people who had been caught up in fashion trends passed on to the Other Side, they became aware of the foolishness of their behavior. They were disappointed in themselves for wasting their time and resources on frivolous Earthly things when they found out that *people and family were so much more important than things*.

CHAPTER 33

History, Journals, and Marvels to Come

On the Other Side, words are not required for clear understanding because all thoughts and intentions are known and understood with clarity.

Words that have been spoken, however, do not just disappear into the air; they remain and can be tuned into and understood. I believe I could have heard anything from the Beatitudes to the Gettysburg Address just as if I were there when they were first uttered. All words are still present if the time is right to tune into them. As I realized that all thoughts, words, and deeds are waiting for review on the Other Side, I wished I could call back all the words I had spoken in harshness.

New Dimensions of Understanding

Everything I saw over there was communicated to me with clear understanding. Some scenes were separate from others and some were connected, although it was as if they were all still present. Time has a different dimension in the spiritual realm. Describing it as a fourth dimension seems inadequate. If Einstein gave us four dimensions of space and time in his theories of relativity, then I would call this the fifth dimension. I have learned since my near death experience that a physicist friend of mine, who has done research in this area, calls the fifth dimension the *eternity domain*. Also, I have learned that he has scientific evidence that space and time are Earthly limitations.

The Importance of Journals

I wanted to communicate to my posterity. I realized it would have been valuable to have left them a written account of what I had learned during Earth life. But now I couldn't—I didn't have my body anymore.

In the spiritual sphere, I saw and felt the importance of writing in diaries or journals and keeping track of family history. I realized keenly that as a person grows and develops in life, it is important to leave a written account of the lessons we learn through life so that others who follow may benefit from our experiences. I understood the importance of learning from the personal experiences of others.

The difficulty and yet the importance of conveying to posterity the lessons learned during Earth life was profoundly impressed upon my mind! Also, I knew that journals and family history accounts could be visible gifts of love for posterity to read. Through them people could get to know their ancestors and have an understanding of who they were and what they believed.

Family history and journals could make it possible for posterity to continue worthwhile traditions, develop their own family traditions, and have a better chance to avoid pitfalls that may have plagued other family members before them.

During Earth life, I had occasionally written in journals, but I didn't keep it up. I had many excuses and believed my journals would not be interesting to anyone. However, I saw that someday some of my posterity—my children's children and their children—would be interested in reading my journals and their family history. They would want to know about me, their great-great-grandmother, who had lived before them during Earth life.

Leaving a Gift in Writing—a Family History

Previously, I had thought of myself as a daughter, granddaughter, and great-granddaughter, but now I realized I would also be a great-grandmother and great-great-grandmother, and so on. I had never really thought about *posterity*, other than my grandchildren who were already born, until I had this glimpse of them. Then I knew the importance of leaving them a written account of their family history. I had an overwhelming desire to communicate to them, to let them know that I cared.

As I thought of the love and concern I had for my previously unknown future family members, they did not seem too distant or too many to know and love. Love is limitless and has no bounds.

119

Thinking about the importance of family journals, I knew that the tone of the messages within them needed to be positive and upbeat—not writings that might hurt or embarrass another person, or things that someone might decide to tear up and throw away. They needed to be uplifting, yet true.

It became evident how much power there is in saying good things about others and keeping a record of the highlights of life, yet not disregarding challenges or pitfalls. I realized the need of emphasizing messages such as to "keep on keeping on," to look for blessings and to record miracles. It was also important to keep the writings focused on overcoming and learning so that posterity could look back and grow from what was shared with them.

There was great value, I now knew, in writing and sharing messages of hope and encouragement—nuggets of knowledge and wisdom learned from the journey of life.

Some people have suggested writing down bad experiences, even venomous words and the worst of feelings; but for every action, even writing down feelings, there is absolutely a reaction. Forgiving, letting go, and loving unconditionally are worthwhile thoughts and actions that will be multiplied for the good of all concerned, especially when recording events and feelings in journals. *Words are powerful!*

Heavenly Stress-Reducers

My thoughts expanded with an increased awareness of many people living on Earth during my lifetime and how they suffered under burdens of stress unique to our period of the world's ongoing history. I became aware of many things that could decrease stress, such as overcoming negative patterns of *reacting* to other people with anger, and following wise counsel as taught in scriptures such as "judge not that ye be not judged." I knew that the more scriptural teachings were followed, the more stress would be relieved.

I also knew that during Earth life, being empathetic and less easily offended adds to peace of mind which will extend to the Other Side.

Present and Future

My view did not end with the past or present; the panorama continued into the future. I recall that it seemed humorous to me that I once thought the present was so advanced, technologically and otherwise, because it is still in the "dark ages" compared to what will be forthcoming in the future.

I was truly inspired to realize how Earth knowledge and technology will continue to advance and expand. For instance, great discoveries and improvements will be made in what is considered "conventional" medical treatments. Alternate fields of healing will be more accepted and there will be faster, more accurate diagnostic techniques and treatments. Other technological advances, I learned, would dwarf what I knew during my Earth life.

My feelings about so many things were changed from seeing history happen. Again, it was like seeing puzzle pieces that had been randomly scattered finally fit together.

Phases of History

I know we are progressing from one phase of history to another, from the past, through the present and into the future. I am extremely grateful that I was allowed to come back to Earth and see some of these futuristic, remarkable things unfold. Having a better perspective helps me to understand more of what is taking place. It is fascinating to know that revolutionary technologies and marvelous inventions are coming, such as improved, new medical advances for maintaining health, outwitting disease, and *faster*, more *accurate* diagnostic techniques.

Some have already come about. It has been a marvelous experience to watch some of the things unfold that spark memories of being on the Other Side. Medical science has done almost unbelievable things, but there is yet much more to come, such as wondrous alternative-medical cures, and other natural remedies and healing discoveries for the body.

The body is a truly miraculous gift of the Creator.

121

CHAPTER 34

Eternal Beauty Secrets

Abruptly, my view of the scenes and the panorama of the history of Earth ended and the spirit world was again revealed. I was surprised as I realized more about God's ever-present and observable love. Feeling His love was glorious and beautiful—a beauty that encompassed everything and everyone in my view.

It is difficult to describe the beauty of the people I saw and felt in the spiritual sphere; it was incredible. I am not talking about outer beauty, but a loveliness that came from deep within and enhanced physical features.

This inner radiance had nothing to do with age. In fact, age itself was interesting; it seemed to me that everyone I saw or of whom I was aware was at their ideal age although there were those who seemed older and those who seemed younger. I do not believe those who appeared older were actually older spirits; perhaps they looked that way for my view.

Goodness Is Beauty

In Earth life, youth and beauty had seemed so connected. On the Other Side, I was surprised that two spirits who were among the most attractive were a man and a woman who looked older to me. Their faces were creased with wrinkles and I realized that each of their wrinkles was a visual testament of the lives they had led in mortality.

My understanding was opened and I became aware of the sorrows and trials this man and woman had withstood in life. Each wrinkle seemed to be a badge of valor that stood for their righteous concerns, a crisis, or an ongoing struggle they had weathered with success. Each line seemed to tell a story; every action, every thought, pain, and concern were known. They were beautiful people because of their mercy, compassion, patience, and love for others. I was awed because I had never considered wrinkles in the face as attractive, but they were to me now, as I understood what these people had gone through, and knew of their tears and pleas to God for mercy and help for others.

Then I began noticing other faces more carefully. There were some who were marred by the lines in their faces. Since every action and thought was known, I knew that many of these lines had been formed by frowning, scowling, excessive anger, and mean-spiritedness. Their faces reflected their former enjoyment of gloating, hurting, and taking advantage of others while on Earth. These choices were now causing them anguish and sorrow.

The Beauty Within

What a contrast! Suddenly I understood a great truth about beauty. On Earth, I believed beauty came from youth and flawless features. In the spirit world, it became obvious that beauty is created from loving, caring, charitable thinking and actions—by endurance through trials with good attitudes. It came from within and was manifested in the outer appearance.

I saw many who had been considered plain and homely on Earth accepted among the most lovely, according to the way they had conducted themselves while in mortality. I saw that those who had an illusion of beauty while in mortality would be seen by eyes of new understanding on the Other Side. They would be perceived from every angle. They had a special radiance if they had conducted themselves well while in their Earthly life.

All Good Deeds Are Rewarded

My concept of beauty was greatly expanded to include my view of each individual as a whole person with their inner self and their outer beauty radiating a loving countenance, or a lack of it. Looks from an Earthly perspective were insignificant in the afterlife.

I received the marvelous knowledge that all good thoughts and deeds are eventually rewarded and add to a person's eternal, radiating countenance.

CHAPTER 35

Caring Relationships Do Not End at Death

It was impressed upon me that heavenly, caring relationships begin on Earth and do not end at death. In fact, they can be stronger and even more special on the Other Side.

I observed people of all shapes and sizes, ages and ethnicities. I remained me—a mother who greatly cared about her family. I was a daughter concerned about her mother, and I knew that relationships of family and friends continue and we can be reunited with our loved ones who have passed on.

Suddenly I felt very alone. My marriage on Earth had not worked out. I felt no blame or unkind feelings; in fact I had a new understanding and sorrow for our differences and problems. I was sorry for any of my wrong actions or reactions, yet we were not right for each other.

However, I knew that friendship, companionship, and the relationships between men and women can be special— more than I had ever realized before. This magnified my loneliness and my desire for another chance at Earth life to find a companion so that we might enjoy the journey of life together.

My thoughts were immediately filled with the all-encompassing love from God. As I rejoiced and felt encircled in His love, I knew that the added love of the companion I desired would have been an extra joy because God's love is so great it dissolved all my feelings that I was unloved.

I experienced a sharp awareness of an increased love and caring for my family and friends. My concern wasn't only for those people with whom I now felt ties, but also for people I had hardly known, or had not previously known who were connected to me.

Happy Homecoming or Lost Blessings

I became aware of many of my ancestors including some I had heard about as a child. The knowledge came to me that if we have met the challenges in life and then died (that is, if our arrival on the Other Side is not due to our own misguided actions) we are received in an attitude of homecoming. We are greeted with a great outpouring of love from those on the Other Side who have been anxiously watching and who have been eager for us to succeed on Earth in our mortal school. Ancestors and posterity are concerned for our success during our Earth life and exist in a sphere close to us even though we cannot see them with our mortal eyes. Our ancestors love and care for us and we love them. *We are important to each other.*

However, those who do something to cause their own death—commit suicide, or give up and regrettably will themselves to die when it's not their time, as I did—*may* have feelings of real sadness for blessings that were lost by their own actions. Also, there *may* be a turning away of loved ones, posterity and ancestors whom we let down. Especially ancestors who had endured difficulties, suffered, and sacrificed for their posterity, they *may* turn away rather than welcome someone's untimely arrival on the Other Side. Only God can judge. Only God knows the true intent of the heart.

Ancestors Are Great Supporters

There were no greater supporters, I realized, than my ancestors who had paved my way with their actions and their very lives. I remember that there were many—some were dressed in angelic white robes and others in clothing that seemed appropriate for differing periods of history. I was aware that they could appear to me in different attire if it would help my understanding.

Their manner of dress was not impressed on my mind as vividly as was my discomfort in being with them; I wanted to retreat from their presence. Their exact words were not clear but I understood that they wanted to convey definite messages of love and concern. They were sad that I had given up. I knew that most of them had endured physical and emotional tragedies on Earth and yet they did not give up. Knowing this, I felt great sorrow that I had not done better with my Earth time. These feelings of regret were woven like threads through my entire experience on the Other Side.

Ancestral Cheerleaders

My ancestors cared about the decisions I made, my actions, and my happiness. Their attitudes could best be described as mental and spiritual cheerleaders. I learned that there are many people interested in each of our lives—more than I ever imagined. As I realized my importance to them, I knew how disappointed they were when I cheated myself by willing myself to die instead of making the most of my opportunities.

While I was on the Other Side, I was aware that when I was alive on Earth and influenced by anger, false pride, or sin, I repelled rather than attracted special spiritual blessings. I saw that when I was tempted to give up on life, to think and act contrary to God's laws, I was vulnerable to influence by spirits who desired my failure, depression, and sadness. Those dark spirits found satisfaction when I wandered from my goals in life and forfeited peace of mind on the Other Side. I knew they were *real* and as desirous of my failure as my spiritual and ancestral cheerleaders were of my success.

Getting Rid of the Influence of Dark Spirits

The realization came to me that these darker spirits were unable to reach me when I chose positive, uplifting thoughts and activities—especially when I prayed, or read scriptures and pondered their spiritual messages! I had my freedom to choose what to think and what to do, and God was there to help me with my choices. *Dark spirits have limitations and could have only influenced my thoughts if I permitted them to.*

Knowing that thoughts create attitudes and then produce actions, I learned the importance of controlling thoughts. I recognized wrongful patterns such as envy, anger, and hurtful actions for what they had been—dangers to my lasting happiness.

Spiritual Showers

As I wondered how to combat the efforts of dark spirits, I thought about comparing a cleansing shower with reading and pondering scriptures.

Scripture study was like a spiritual shower because it caused the dark spirits to disappear; they recoiled in the presence of Godly things. I could have felt spiritually clean and more receptive to inspiration by studying great eternal truths, more capable of living a Godlike life, and more able to take part in God's Grand Plan.

It was now clear to me that there are many truths and answers in scriptures and other Great Books of Holy Writings which could have given me a more righteous perspective and a more abundant life. The path for a life of lasting peace is detailed there. The wisdom, for example, found in the Sermon on the Mount or Beatitudes (Matthew 5:1-12) and in Scriptures such as this one: "Inasmuch as ye have done it unto one of the least of these my brethren, ye have done it unto me" (Matthew 25:40).

While I was on the Other Side, I was shown vivid scenes that reinforced the importance of living our lives in accord with Scriptures such as, "If ye love me, keep my commandments." (John 14:15) and "In my Father's house are many mansions: if it were not so, I would have told you. I go to prepare a place for you" (John 14:2).

Another vivid scene I recall was of the incident in Matthew where someone asked Jesus: "Teacher, which is the greatest commandment in the Law?"

Jesus replied: "'Love the Lord your God with all your heart and with all your soul and with all your mind.'[a] 38 This is the first and greatest commandment. 39 And the second is like it: 'Love your neighbor as yourself.'[b] 40 All the Law and the Prophets hang on these two commandments" (Matthew 22:36-40).

It is hard to put into words, but I essentially saw the truth of this passage in scenes that were so vivid and penetrating that I feel they are now forever engraved on my heart and soul.

Stepping Stones to Wisdom

I also realized these books could not give guidance if they were not read! I knew that reading them, studying them prayerfully, and pondering them, would allow knowledge to enter the mind and open the channel of inspiration and understanding for a higher way of living that causes dark spirits to flee. Now I understood how *literally true, yet understated the scriptures are.*

As I understood the wisdom and eternal success principles found in the scriptures and how powerful they were, all the thousands of books written to help everyone come to the same conclusions seemed irrelevant. Most of them would not be necessary if scriptures were really *studied, understood,* and *applied* in our lives. However, I also realized that the myriad of books and self-improvement courses can be stepping-stones leading to better understanding and application of the teachings of the Great Books—knowledge of eternal truths help us overcome the stumbling blocks in the journey of life.

Reaping Miraculous Results

From my experience on the Other Side, I learned many things. One conclusion I reached is that life is similar to a treasure chest filled with vast treasures, for here and for heaven, but it has a big lock on it. Holding grudges, using harsh words, running from life and oneself by using drugs or alcohol and avoiding problems only makes the lock stronger.

There are "Grand Keys" to opening the lock that I learned. They are: *striving to be slow to anger, being quick to forgive, and seeking heavenly help by communicating with God through sincere prayer.*

In addition, I know that problems can be solved by believing in miracles, expecting miracles, and helping to create miraculous results for someone else. All such miracles reap eternal rewards.

Prayer and Surroundings

Prayer is a special time. After my experience on the Other Side, as I now pray, I mentally picture God in my mind as a real, loving, personable, all-wise, all-powerful, and all-knowing God who wants me to be grateful for what I have.

As I kneel to pray in the morning, I feel it is helpful for me to take a few moments and call to mind those whom the Lord would have me be mindful of that day. By being more aware of others' needs, I feel more in tune with God. When I am more in harmony with His desired outcome of my day, I know I am more apt to have my prayers answered favorably and to receive His peace.

Also, I prefer to get in a reverent physical and spiritual setting when I can. I do not delay my prayers, though, just because I am not in the right place or I don't look right. He listens and can hear, no matter how or where someone prays to Him. His love is extended to all, regardless of situation and apparel. Prayers are answered according to His own timetable.

When I prepare myself before praying, I feel more respectful. God is as real as any other being—certainly more special than anyone I might meet in Earth life. Just as I comb my hair and straighten my appearance before opening the door to a friend or stranger, I want to do so before opening a dialogue with the most important being in my life. Prayer time can be anytime, anywhere, but I like to keep in mind with whom I am conversing, and make it special whenever I can.

My new attitude has to do with the reverence and respect I feel for Him since I have come to know Him better. Remembering the scripture that tells of Moses approaching the burning bush, the voice told him to remove his shoes, for the ground on which he stood was holy. For me now, I remind myself that prayer time is holy time, and I want to be even more respectful than I would talking with any other person.

Usually, I want to tell Him how much I sincerely appreciate what I have been given, the blessings I've received, and prayers that have been answered. It is important to thank Him for the gifts He has given before I ask for more.

It is not necessary to use eloquent speech when I pray, because I know God is understanding and knows the intent of my heart. It is important to pray in the manner I feel is comfortable and appropriate. When I was on the Other Side, I learned that He wants to hear from me—and from all of us. When I think of prayer as a two-way communication, it becomes easier to pray.

Whisperings of the Spirit

There are moments when the veil seems to draw back and memories from the Other Side return. These experiences are similar to walking into a room filled with dear and familiar people and experiences. Wondering how

I could have ever forgotten some of them, I realize I didn't really forget. They are still there, but the pressures of day-to-day living pushed them to the back of my memory.

It is enjoyable when someone says something that refreshes my memory of scenes and feelings from the Other Side, and I remember how wondrously whole the purpose and plan of life really is. The combined feelings of love, connections to people, nature, knowledge about forgiveness and the desire to forgive others quickly well up within me. I re-experience some of the glorious feelings about life I felt then and deep gratitude for my mortal existence.

My love for others expanded when I learned the Great Eternal Truth that each person is a unique individual with definite, differing personalities; that we always will be known by and unconditionally loved by God. Through whisperings of the Spirit, we can all know that we have always been uniquely us even before we were born. We didn't just begin with life on Earth. We can also know that our identity continues after Earth life—we don't stop being us at death.

Helping Others Helps Me

When I am feeling stressed or not feeling as mentally "up" as I would like, I usually call someone who I know needs help. I know it does *not* help to call someone to complain about life or to criticize. A technique I have found that works wonders is to call someone with cheerful, good news or to help someone else have an "up" day. Helping someone else, usually helps me.

Also, as I share my experience with others in a way that helps them, it helps me to relive it and remember what I learned from it. Remembering the significance and reality of what I experienced continues to help me here.

For several years, my mother and several others, urged me to publish my experiences, but I hesitated. Then I began receiving letters and calls from people telling me of the positive differences my story had made in the lives of those with whom I had shared; they wanted their own loved ones to know about it, too.

Ultimately, I gathered my courage and decided it was time to speak up more actively. Sometimes I speak on a one-to-one basis and other times with groups, as I feel prompted. Several times on an airplane the feeling has come to me that I must tell the person next to me a portion of my story.

When I get such feelings, they grow until I feel compelled to speak up. Then I begin a casual conversation and generally, with the other person's first few words, I learn why I felt impressed to speak to them. As I mentioned before, in many of life's situations, God uses people (whenever they are willing) to answer the prayers of others.

When Others Need Help

Since returning from the Other Side, there have been times that miraculous episodes have occurred when I told my story to strangers. Some needed a push to go to the dentist, others were suffering from an ailment I accurately pinpointed which they were then able to overcome by seeking proper help.

Sometimes the person was feeling depressed or suicidal, and later I learned that they made changes in their lives and were doing better. I was glad our paths crossed when they did and I was able to help.

A Gift of Empathy

Upon returning to Earth life, with the new, expanded knowledge I had gained, I felt more empathetic toward others. I treasure this empathy as a gift. When I look at others' faces and countenances now, whether I am speaking to an audience, interacting with someone in a restaurant, sitting next to a stranger on an airplane or almost anywhere, I seem intuitively to discern the pain and joy that the people around me have experienced in their lives.

Sensing their inner beauty, struggles, and sincerity or lack thereof, I begin to *feel* much about them. When I would look into people's eyes and see their expressions, I understood them better and become aware of many of their needs, wants, fears, pains, and struggles.

CHAPTER 36

Lasting Peace of Mind

It was surprising to learn how much God loves and appreciates the sincere and devout of all faiths who seek to better themselves and aid humanity. The love of God abounds for all—He is no respecter of persons of one over another. Never before had I felt so connected with all people and all religions as I did when I realized the extent of His love. He has such rich rewards waiting for those who sincerely strive to follow Him.

I wondered why there were so many religions on Earth, and I wondered about their greatly varying teachings, scriptures, and interpretations of them. It was shown to me that some teachings in different religions in the world are nearer to God's truths than others. Those that are closest are generally found in some form in all religions; for example, treating others as we would have them treat us. I was keenly aware that we are all at our own level of spiritual beliefs and at our own level of ability to live by religious teachings. I had a bright awareness that God is pleased with all those who strive for righteousness.

Hungering and Thirsting for Righteousness

As people fervently and sincerely seek to know the truth and to live God's laws, He is pleased, and their spiritual selves are expanded. They become capable of receiving more inspiration, knowledge, and truth; *they reap blessings*. I knew that the more people apply the knowledge and inspiration they are given, the more they can receive.

I was also shown that there were many people who were complacent and unwisely satisfied with what they believe. Yet I was aware that there were vast numbers of people sincerely striving to gain answers to life's questions and knowledge of Eternal Truths. Driven by a great hunger and thirst for righteousness, they sample the teachings of many religions of the world. Seeking to drink from a "living well," they rightly search until they find the religion that gives them guidance and inner peace.

These sincere people look for the religion they believe is right for them and that fulfills their quest for knowledge about their own true purpose for living.

Nothing Is Too Small for God's Concern

My wonderment continued as I realized how all-knowing God is. No care or problem is too small for Him to know everything about it.

I realized that God offers a peace beyond comprehension or description, an eternal peace of mind! I had never even imagined that God was so all-knowing. As my understanding was opened, I knew He is fully aware of everyone's problems, temptations, and sorrows. He is aware of sincerity, righteous sacrifices, and the intent of each heart as His children strive to live by His commandments.

My soul was filled with love and appreciation for the sincere believers of all the world's religions. I understood that God's Holy Words offer a lasting peace beyond worldly description for all. The greatest and most lasting peace of mind for Earth life and the Other Side is offered to all humanity by God.

CHAPTER 37

Prayer, Promptings, and Whisperings of the Spirit

Next, I saw and became aware of many aspects of prayer and how important it is to pray. Learning that prayer truly is a conversation with God, I realized that He wanted to hear from me and to communicate with me. I then knew the importance of expressing gratitude and appreciation for all my blessings—from small things to great miracles.

Connecting to Heavenly Power

Feeling remorse that I had taken for granted many special blessings, I now saw my life in its proper perspective. I knew that electricity was powerful and capable of mighty accomplishments when something is connected to it. But I saw that being connected to heavenly power in prayer is an infinitely greater power that draws from a "heavenly treasury." I knew that miracles are possible and happen much more frequently than acknowledged on Earth.

During my Earth life, I had not adequately realized this amazing source of power. Many times I prayed from habit or because I needed something in particular. But at this point, I saw prayer, silent and spoken, as a two-way communication with someone I loved and respected, who loved me and had the power to bless me for my good. In my life review, I saw that many of my prayers had been granted, and I felt remorse that I had not recognized and expressed appreciation for my blessings.

Knowledge was given to me about unanswered prayers and how they had been for my benefit. I understood the importance of God's timing in the context of my whole life, rather than my own desire to have everything right now. Also, I more fully realized the great importance of doing what I could with what I had and appreciating it, rather than concentrating on and lamenting over what I did not have.

My mind was quickened with the knowledge that there were answers to prayers and blessings I had received where I had falsely given the credit to "coincidence," instead of giving thanks to God in all things.

Visualizing a Personal God

Knowledge was given to me about the importance of praying regularly and thinking of God as a person. There were times when I used to pray and my mind would wander because I did not have a clear understanding and mental picture of God. I was thrilled to know that He is an actual Being who has feelings and that He loves me. This was not just some cloud I was speaking to when I knelt in prayer. I discovered He is much more knowledgeable, understanding, and loving than any other person I could ever imagine knowing.

Receiving Answers to Prayers

My awareness was opened to some of the many things involved in receiving answers to prayers, such as the sincerity of mind and heart and the *readiness* of the person to receive the requested help asked for. Sometimes an answer to a prayer to have a burden removed comes in the form of strength to carry it rather than a miracle to take the burden or problem away.

Also, I saw the definite connection between the likelihood of receiving mercy and help requested to the mercy and help the person praying has given others. Knowledge was given me that God usually uses willing people to answer others' prayers. I became aware that our prayers are more apt to be answered when we ask and respond positively to the questions *"Whose burden could I lighten today as I ask God to help ease mine? Who is waiting to hear from me?* **With wisdom**, *whose pain could I ease with loving words or deeds so I could then ask with a clear conscience for my prayer to be answered?"*

God is keenly aware of everyone's prayers. It is unproductive to ask Him to answer our prayers when we deliberately ignore the needs of those we ought to be mindful of—especially elderly parents and grandparents who wait to hear or need help from children and loved ones.

Scenes came to my mind of people on Earth who were preoccupied with their babies and other children to the extent that they neglected aging

135

parents and grandparents who had expended their time, strength, and means caring for them when they were young.

As the years rolled by, some of the elderly parents in the scenes I viewed became so weak that they were no longer able to care for themselves. They needed attention from their children and grandchildren. Because they felt lost and forgotten, they gave up and simply waited to die. What a difference a visit, a phone call, or a card would have made to them. They waited day after day with no contact from even their closest loved ones—those on whom they had spent their own time and resources.

Watching and hearing older parents and grandparents praying and asking God to ease their burdens and loneliness made me feel great sadness for all concerned. I was aware that many promptings to their children to make those requested calls or visits were sadly unheeded. Yet, the children and grandchildren were asking God to answer their own prayers while they were oblivious to those whose prayers *they* could so easily answer.

Take Time to Listen to the Whisperings of the Spirit

I learned that while praying to God, expressing gratitude, and asking for blessings, it is also very important to pause and take time to listen to *promptings* that may come as *whisperings* from the Holy Spirit. Promptings may be blocked by becoming too caught up in "asking." When we take time to *listen* we can receive the inspiration, promptings, and guidance that brings peace beyond measure.

Continually asking for blessings, I realized, without giving sincere thanks, is like a child asking a parent for more and more without taking time to give thanks and appreciation for what has already been received. God wants to receive thanks as do Earthly parents.

I Longed to Return to My Body

Vividly aware of how my decisions and actions could so personally affect the lives of others and myself, I longed for the chance to come back and make right what I could; to progress and grow through life and not run from it. I wanted to come back and change whatever ill effects my death would cause others, and to use my Earth time more effectively.

Although I had not actually committed suicide, I had completely surrendered my life, willing myself to die, and God had granted my desire. Now, in this sphere, the implications of my choices were clear. Starkly apparent were things that I wanted to do on Earth that I had not done and could have done. Thoughts of my family came again to my mind and I wanted to tell them what I had learned about the Other Side.

Amazing Heavenly Answers Discovered

Also, I wanted to tell others who were looking for hope about the heavenly answers to problems on Earth that I had discovered. I wanted to shout the real value of life on Earth and the foolishness of trying to cut life short to escape problems and physical discomforts.

When I saw things in the proper perspective, I wanted to live even in an aching, mortal body. Every part of my mind, heart, and spirit begged to have another chance to go back to the Earthly sphere. Feelings of "if only" were tormenting me.

I was struck with the knowledge that in Earth life, it was not how physically impaired one is that matters or what physical abilities were gone; rather, it was how one used what was left. I was desperately willing to be once again shackled with my physical limitations.

In the spiritual sphere, I was free from physical pain for the first time in many long years, yet the emotional anguish I was feeling was many times worse than the physical pain I'd had when I was alive. I wanted to escape this spiritual misery even more than I had wanted to escape my physical pain.

Unhappily, I felt that asking to return was useless. I had lived my life. I had had the chance to live or die and had chosen to die. I had prayed for death and here it was. It seemed futile to request another chance, yet I couldn't stop myself. The more I thought about the opportunities I had let slip past me, the more I wanted to be allowed to return.

CHAPTER 38

Drawn Back into My Earthly Body

The Truth about a Gold-Crowned Tooth

While on the Other Side, suddenly, I saw in my mind's eye a large image of one of my gold-crowned teeth. I'd had the crown for over fifteen years and knew exactly which tooth this was in the upper right quadrant. During all those years I had not given that tooth any thought because it had not given me any pain. I had a thorough dental checkup not long before this experience, and all my teeth checked out fine. Nevertheless, God revealed to me that it was a major source of many of my health problems and an important part of the answer to recovering my physical health.

A Gift of Knowledge

The dangers and health problems caused by amalgam fillings (which are 50% mercury) was also revealed to me. Before this experience, I did not know that such a simple thing as a tooth could cause or contribute to so much damage to health. This vivid and complete gift of knowledge about my tooth played a vital part in the possibility that I could live again in my physical body, although I did not know why at that instant.

Mortally Alive Again

Just as suddenly as it had appeared, the tooth vanished. Then, without warning, I was suddenly, quickly drawn back into my body. Still leaning forward toward the inside of the tub, I stared at the bottom of the bathtub for a while, realizing that miraculously I was back on Earth. I began trying to push myself up from the edge of the tub. Slowly, I made my body move. My fingers moved; I gradually moved my hands and I touched my face. I was solid, mortally alive again!

Turning my head, I noted with amazement that I could only see what was in my normal field of vision. The "everywhere at once" vision I'd had in the spirit world was gone.

I was not that wispy being anymore. I had a new awareness that this Earth world is not actually the *real* world.

A Return to Earth Life

Immediately, I was aware of physical pain; I ached throughout my whole body. There were sharp pains in my arms, legs, hands, and feet, and I had very little strength. My weakness was so profound that it made gravity seem powerful and oppressive. But I didn't care. I had no desire to exchange my situation of pain and sickness for that light, floaty, pain-free existence. *I was after all being given another chance at life!*

The anguish was gone; my agony of spirit was over. Kneeling shakily and leaning on the tub, I felt the glorious thrill of once again being alive and on the Earth. My pleas to return to Earth life had been granted. Gratitude welled up inside of me. Joy and relief overwhelmed me. I was overjoyed to be where I was; even grateful to feel exhausted, to feel my body's pain, and to feel ill.

I tried to get back into bed and found that I couldn't walk; even crawling was difficult. The effort was exhausting because I was so weak and my movements were slow. But all the way I kept thinking, "I can move my body. I am alive!"

I then somehow managed to drag my exhausted body back into bed.

Gratitude beyond Expression

Uncertain as to how long I had been on the Other Side, I was overjoyed to have returned. The gratitude I felt was beyond my ability to express. Thinking of how, only a short time before, I was wishing for release from my Earthly existence, now I was ecstatic to have returned to life in any physical condition.

Even though I was ill, I now knew that being alive was a great blessing. I was determined to stop putting limitations on my body by thinking negative thoughts about my health. My body was precious and priceless no matter what it looked like or how ill it was.

No Clocks Needed on the Other Side

Managing to get back into bed, Earth life seemed to be the *foreign* sphere where time and clocks were odd. The Other Side was the natural sphere where no clocks were needed. There I experienced a dimension of time where everything was *now*—where a person's intent of the heart and words were not misinterpreted, and where all truth was known. That was the *real* sphere.

Earth Time Is Precious

Directly after my experience on the Other Side, with my new knowledge of the value of time, I thought that I would never again watch television or sit for hours in a movie theater. I did not want to waste one precious moment of my life.

Still, I do understand the need for keeping a balance between worthwhile goals and needed leisure time; but I think people need to be careful of the quantity and quality. Personally, I want the benefits of surrounding myself with inspirational and educational things rather than detrimental, destructive words or scenes.

Back for How Long?

Knowing the significance of returning to Earth life, though, and being thrilled that I could speak again, I said aloud, "I am back, I am really back." Tears of joy spilled down my cheeks. Then concerns struck me.

I'm back, but for how long?

How long will I be given to do the things I want to do in Earth life?

How long will I have to put into practice the perspectives that I gained?

No answer came to me. Knowing that I had no guarantees, no idea of the length of time I was being given, I knew I had to make every moment count. Being anxious to get busy living, I wanted to stand up and start right then. My weakness, though, was such that I could only lie there and contemplate how much I had learned, and how much I wanted to do.

When I felt somewhat stronger, I made my way into the family room where Crystal's foolish video game—my gift to her—was located. She had not been at my home for a couple of days. Slowly, I unhooked the game from the back of the TV set, gathered up the cords and controllers, and hid them away. Then I returned to bed.

The experience I had and the scenes I had viewed which contained symbolic, life-changing messages for me seemed miraculous. Wanting to tell anyone who would listen, I soon told those I trusted the most. My experience was sufficiently personal, though, that I was careful with whom I shared it.

Thoughts Are Powerful

Each hour of the day, I know that I make choices which include deliberately taking control of my thinking or allowing other forces to sway, dictate, or manipulate my thoughts and attitudes. I know that attitudes and desires are formed as a direct result of thoughts held daily in my mind, which then determine what I will accomplish during my life on Earth.

Thoughts are powerful and too valuable to waste!

Between Two Spheres

Throughout the next two weeks, I felt the odd sensation that at anytime, night or day, I could step back into that other sphere, the spirit world. The knowledge I had gained was still fresh in my mind. I could call up the images I had seen at will and re-experience my visit there. Memories of the larger picture of life and life after death impressed upon my mind that Earth life is very temporary.

Although I wanted to be alive with all my heart, I did not want to lose my enlightenment, my knowledge, and the new awareness I had gained. I hoped this bright awareness and access to the Other Side would last the rest of my life, but gradually I felt the spirit world begin to slip away. With my new knowledge, I understood that I could not continue to live on Earth unless I was able to experience life's trials and temptations in a natural way, and little by little I re-entered mortality and felt a part of Earth life once more.

PART THREE

My Life After I Returned to Earth

After having had my life review on the Other Side, which was filled with so many regrets, I knew that the next time I die I want to have Heavenly peace of mind while in God's presence.

However, I was surprised when I had returned to my body with another chance to live. Thinking back over my life review, I realized then, that *anything* I had *previously repented for* while I was alive, was not included in my afterlife review. Mistakes that I had felt terrible about, but had repented of, were *gone*.

I also realized that I had a new purpose for living with an eternal perspective, and the way for me to have this peace of mind would be to share these truths so others can find their own true purpose for living.

With the miracle of another chance to live, I now wanted to savor every moment of life to the fullest. I knew any problems I would encounter were meant for my growth.

CHAPTER 39

The Dentist—My Friend

Among my most vivid memories of the Other Side was the importance of getting that tooth removed. As soon as I could muster enough strength, I made an appointment with my dentist, Dr. Richard Smart, DDS. I told him about my vision of the tooth during my Other Side experience, and requested that he pull it immediately.

"Does it hurt?" he asked.

"No," I said.

"It looks and seems okay," he said positively.

"It may look okay, but it has to come out," I emphatically replied.

He tried to reassure me that I was worrying needlessly. He took an X-ray to appease me. As he showed it to me, he smiled and said, "Joyce, just as I thought, there is nothing wrong with this tooth." He showed me the X-ray, carefully explaining why the tooth was sound.

However, its appearance on the X-ray did not impress me; I absolutely *knew* that the tooth had to be extracted. In my mind, I again saw the tooth—gold crowned,

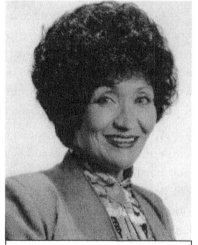

Joyce back from the afterlife and grateful to be alive.

suspended, rotating in front of me. Something was wrong with that tooth and I knew it had to come out. To convince my dentist, I decided to share parts of my experience with him.

He listened carefully and politely, then shook his head slowly, "You know, Joyce, I'm limited to the practice of Western medicine. Nothing I've studied has prepared me professionally to believe I need to take out that tooth. This experience you had just isn't enough for me."

My dentist was a respected professional and he had a way of making his patients feel he was their friend; he treated us with sincerity and concern. He and I had a good rapport, and he could see I was determined to have this particular tooth extracted.

He was so reluctant that in order to pull it he insisted I would need to sign a legal paper releasing him from all liability for extracting what he believed to be a perfectly healthy tooth. After I signed the document, he arranged an appointment with an oral surgeon.

As soon as the tooth was out, the surprised oral surgeon held it out in front of me where we could both obviously see its blackened, decomposed roots which had led to a bad infection up through my jaw and into my sinuses.

Electrical Needles and Pins

As I was leaving his office and for an hour or two afterwards, I felt strange sensations—as though thousands of electrical needles and pins were embedded in the skin all over my body and were working their way out to the surface through all of my pores. It was very uncomfortable. Within twenty-four hours, the mysterious bleeding down the back of my throat stopped as though a tap had been turned off. I was extremely grateful.

A few days after the extraction, I took the tooth back to my regular dentist on a follow-up visit and he examined it closely. He asked if he could cut it in half to observe the interior. I agreed. Silver amalgam filling could be seen beneath the gold. (Until my experience on the Other Side, I didn't know about the severe health problems that could be caused by teeth *or* that silver-mercury amalgam *or* gold and silver in the same tooth could cause health problems.)

He gave the tooth back to me cut into two pieces. He agreed it was a good thing it was out.

A Miraculous Recovery

Within a few days, I went back to see the ear, nose, and throat specialist and took the gold-crowned tooth to show him. He held up half of it at a time with a pair of tweezers and examined it closely. He was usually a quiet man of few words who went in and out of the examination room briskly. Not this time. He looked from the roots of the tooth, to me, then back to the roots of the tooth. He exclaimed emphatically, "Joyce, I never would have gotten you well with that in your mouth."

He told me the roots apparently had been embedded in the sinuses and had been "dissolved" by the infection. The infected tooth was the cause of the internal bleeding from my sinuses as well as the inflammation in my body that had prevented my upper respiratory infections from healing and had become too much for my system to overcome.

Within the next several days, I went to a dentist and had all of my silver amalgam (mercury) fillings removed.

A Gift from God

My delight at receiving that gift from God was soon joined by other blessings. Within two or three weeks the intense pain from my arthritis was almost completely gone. I began recovering miraculously in many ways and my rheumatoid arthritis went into remission.

It is now my belief that teeth with infections, root canals, and especially silver mercury fillings are the *root cause* of many of the illnesses that are almost impossible to diagnose. Over the years, I became more aware of the problems these fillings can cause. I also learned that when these fillings are removed, for their disposal, they have to go into a container that is sent to a *hazardous waste facility*.

I agree with many top holistic medical professionals that there is a great lack of knowledge in dentistry and its connection with our physical health. Warning: We only get the care that the doctor or dentist has had the training and background to provide.

A new trend for doctors, health specialists, and others is towards *functional medicine*. There are benefits and cautions depending on the depth of the practitioner's training.

Without question, I firmly believe that when one has a lingering illness it is wise to seek *holistic* doctors and *holistic* dentists to find the best health solutions.

Also, I believe it is vitally important to obtain thermographic images of the head and body which will show inflammation. The best thermography camera I've found is the Medi-Therm. It is FDA approved. This is not the same type that is used for detecting heat in buildings; this is an entirely different technology.

By using the medical thermographic camera, an *adequately trained* holistic practitioner can usually tell where any inflammation exists in the head or body, which can be a sign of infection or other problems. Numerous times with patients with whom I've worked, it was an infected tooth or multiple teeth that was taking their immune system down.

After the infected teeth were pulled, their health improved, sometimes dramatically, and they had more energy than they'd had in years. Usually, people don't realize to what degree problems with their teeth and gums can affect their general health or even *cause* disease. In fact, my dying and going to the Other Side was caused by a bad tooth.

Despite my own personally transforming near-death experience, I readily admit that I was quite relieved when I first learned of Sam Ziff's 1984 book, *Silver Dental Fillings: The Toxic Time Bomb: Can the Mercury in Your Dental Fillings Poison You?* I no longer felt like a lone wolf in wanting to share the potential dangers of mercury amalgam fillings. Today, 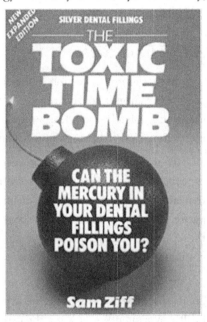 fortunately, the FDA is now acknowledging the potential harm of "mercury-containing" amalgam. The FDA's September 24, 2020 press release, entitled "FDA Issues Recommendations for Certain High-Risk Groups Regarding Mercury-Containing Dental Amalgam," does contain certain qualifiers, but it's an important admission nonetheless, and, moreover, they do explicitly include "people with [a] pre-existing neurological disease such as multiple sclerosis, Alzheimer's disease or Parkinson's disease."

146

There are considerable potential advantages of getting the amalgam fillings removed—not least of which is helping your immune system. Rather than battling the effects of the release of mercury vapor (from eating food, chewing gum, or grinding your teeth), your immune system can concentrate on whatever else your body may be dealing with. If you do have your mercury amalgam filings removed, however, be sure to have the procedure done by a dentist trained in the proper protocol, including using a "dental dam" to prevent any of the mercury particles from sliding down your throat and into your stomach.

People, understandably, often complain to me about the costs of removing amalgam fillings. Depending on the person's health condition, and financial situation, I occasionally feel compelled to remind some of them, "It's cheaper than a funeral!"

When I first returned to Earth life, I still had pain from the failed back surgeries, but my feelings of self-condemnation had been completely replaced with gratitude for life. Also, the appreciation I had acquired for being back in my body made the pain and discomfort bearable.

After struggling with depression for years, I now felt a new purpose for living. I conquered depression and any lingering thoughts of suicide.

I was committed to using the knowledge I had gained to live a better life and to help others. I accepted that I was meant to leave that other world behind, to be back in my physical body, and had a strong desire to live and to meet head on whatever was put in front of me.

What had helped me get through life so far was prayers, miracles, *sleep learning*, determined willpower and positive affirmations. However, it was not until my near-death experience that I realized and understood that my purpose for living was working *through* problems rather than giving up because of them.

I discovered that suicide is not the answer, and what is important is to be grateful, loving, kind, forgiving, and merciful.

These things feed the human soul, and as you learn how to draw on the powers of heaven in the pages ahead you will find many additional answers for your own earthly challenges.

Still, there were many challenges ahead in my own life.

CHAPTER 40

A Heavenly Perspective

Shortly after coming back, I remember wishing I could grab a megaphone and shout my message from the tallest building. I enthusiastically told several people close to me about it. However, as I carefully pondered the entire occurrence I began to realize I had mixed feelings about sharing it—having a "Near Death Experience" was not a subject openly discussed at the time. Also, the experience felt sacred and personal to me. This was the 1980s, whereas today these experiences are much more common and openly shared. In fact, I still receive regular requests to speak to groups about my experience.

Nevertheless, I was extremely excited about returning to Earth's mortal sphere, and part of me wanted to tell everyone what I had learned: *Heavenly answers to Earthly challenges are available for all and so is the knowledge that permits us to be certain of enjoying the Other Side when we get there.*

When another individual's need to hear about my experience on the Other Side became apparent, I shared it with assurance. At that time, I felt I was one of the most confident people on Earth. I knew who I was: *a child of God!* For quite awhile after my experience, I didn't think I'd ever fear being in the presence of other people again.

Gradually though, as time passed, my self-confidence in speaking about my experience began to dim. As I settled back into Earth life, my experience and the lessons I had learned began to slip to the back of my mind rather than being the focus of my daily attention .

Seeing Trials as Heavenly Stepping Stones

During the first few weeks after my return I was grateful for each problem awaiting me, because I knew of the benefits I could receive when I overcame them. By understanding problems in their proper eternal perspective, I realized that each difficult experience, well lived with sincere intentions, was like a jewel on a crown. Its message would sparkle with rewards for having triumphed and passed through a refiner's fire. I knew that progressing through life would be enormously easier if I remembered to evaluate events from the eternal perspective.

The attitude I took in any given situation was my choice! With my new eternal outlook at that time, I was able to see life's experiences in a different way. Trials were blessings, and I wanted to make it through them with the right attitude.

Do I Want Sympathy or Results?

It was clear that I had wasted a lot of time before my experience on the Other Side thinking, "Why me? Why did this happen to me?" Thoughts of "Why me?" or "Why now?" solve nothing and can lead to depression. Additionally, they waste valuable time and stop possible solutions that could have come to mind. It would be as if my coat caught on fire and I yelled "Why me?" as I wrung my hands while it burned rather than dousing the flames while they were still small. If I act, rather than ask "why me?" I can put out the "fire" and be grateful it wasn't worse. Then I can practice "fire prevention" in the future. Handling problems in this manner helps me find solutions rather than waste time uselessly seeking answers that will not be revealed until I view things from the perspective of the Other Side .

CHAPTER 41

A Career-Changing Lawsuit

Love came into my life and I married retired air force major Earl Brown in December of 1983. We met and married while he was President of Producer's Livestock Marketing. Our future looked bright. He was a widower and had a very special family. Interestingly, I still think of some of them every year on their birthdays. I also remember seeing a picture of Earl when he was in the service with the chest of his uniform covered in medals. He served in World War II, the Korean War, and Vietnam.

Although there were many positives, unexpectedly, in the spring of 1984, Earl had a major heart attack which brought on serious health problems and great challenges. The doctors said that he only had weeks to live and could die of a major heart attack at any time.

Making sure he got the care and treatments he needed, it critically divided my time as a caregiver and busy professional business owner.

Utilizing holistic health care treatments, he totally improved—so much so that he went back to work for the place where he had retired.

The Power of Thoughts

Realizing the rewards to be received by forgiving others, I wanted to forgive everyone for everything. By knowing that offenses to me could be opportunities to forgive others, I later wondered if I might have "issued an unfortunate invitation" for problems after my return to Earth life because of what happened concerning a valuable business contract.

In 1984 and 1985, it became a confusing series of battles to maintain control of the energy conversion contract.

Suddenly, in 1986, I realized that the agents from my alternative energy business, rather than working on my behalf, had instead been trying to cut me out of the profits. They also attempted to eliminate me from the business entirely by trying to replace my long-term government contract with their own.

In early spring of 1986, I also received a letter from a Fortune 500 company recognizing my personal expertise in waste-to-energy, recycling, pollution control and hazardous waste disposal. Furthermore, in this letter they guaranteed performance and financing for my multi-million dollar project. It would produce megawatts of electricity, pollution free, for the power company, replacing coal.

But it was too late.

Unknown to me, my agents had created a new company and my associates and I were excluded from critical and required meetings. Contrary to our contractual agreements, my contract was assigned to this new unknown company and listed as their own asset in legal documents. After they breached my contract, it was finally lost for both of us.

An official representative of the large company I had hired arranged to meet with me and I was expecting to receive a check for $250,000 for the net revenue for the past year. I was surprised and thrilled by this amount since it was, by far, the largest I'd ever received from the project.

Instead, I was shocked when he informed me the corporation was no longer honoring my contract with them. They had closed down the plant, laid off the employees, and made arrangements for a landfill company to take over the facility. However, instead of giving me a check, he told me I would have to retain an attorney and file a lawsuit in order to get my money. I was devastated.

Reluctantly, I retained an attorney, and filed a lawsuit. I did not realize at the time that court cases were full of unexpected delays, that almost always drag out for many years, and that *justice* and *fairness* is most often found only in the dictionary. The large company I was fighting had deep pockets, hired several top attorneys dedicated to this case, and the resulting lawsuit dragged on and on.

After years and extremely high legal fees, and the requirement for me to add additional specialized attorneys who were also to be paid from the settlement, some information surfaced to support my case. A possible settlement was mentioned, but nothing came of it.

The lawsuit also caused stress to my husband. It was demanding more and more of my time and attention to deal with all the details of the case. This just added to the daily challenges.

As I underwent the ordeal of the lawsuit, the stress was causing my muscles to weaken. I also had problems with breathing.

The energy I had to sustain my life was slowly being sapped. The huge financial burdens, the loss of my project, including future income, and the entanglements involved by being in a multi-million dollar lawsuit, caused me to almost crash. I felt devastated.

One day, I collapsed and literally fell to my knees. With heartfelt sorrow, as tears rolled down my cheeks, I prayed harder than ever before for inspiration, guidance, and a miracle. I needed help to get hold of my thinking.

The Wondrous Results of Sleep Learning

Critically, I realized I needed even stronger and more powerfully worded *sleep learning* recordings to help me get control of my thinking, feelings, and actions. I knew that a professional recording studio and special equipment would be required to make this happen.

I called upon all my past experiences and resources to design, create, and develop a more effective Sleep Learning course than any I had used before. It had positive suggestions to help me sleep and to help me handle the stress and to think and feel better.

In 1987, this project became a reality. I produced revolutionary and unique sleep learning recordings using Super-Subliminals™ and Whisper Learning™ with positive affirmations.

After they were produced, listening to them helped me go into a deeper level of sleep, rest more, concentrate better, feel calmer, and have more confidence during even the most stressful situations.

Listening to those positive suggestions helped keep my thoughts and actions more in tune with the principles I had learned on the Other Side for a higher way of living. I used them continuously. Gradually, I made it through hour-by-hour and day-by-day.

The results produced were miraculous. Because the courses were unique and produced results, I had requests from people who wanted to purchase them and offers from others who wanted to market them. But I was trapped in a legal web and could not fill the requests at that time. The lost revenues for the unfilled orders was considerable.

Since then I have transferred these recordings to digital to make them compatible with present day technology and available to others. They are now available for a donation (you choose the amount) on my website: https://hopedr.org

Attorneys Everywhere

The corporation I was up against had numerous attorneys and seemed to have almost unlimited time and funds for a legal battle. The intrigue could fill a book of its own. Attorneys were everywhere, on both sides of this issue, with corresponding legal expenses. I remembered that directly after my return from the Other Side, I had wanted an opportunity to forgive and it came abundantly. For a time, my tears flowed with thoughts of "could-have-beens" and "should-have-beens" that my original contract would have produced for all concerned had it been honored. According to expert witnesses' figures as well as our own, I had lost a fortune.

With exceptional attorneys, witnesses, and evidence that seemed overwhelmingly in my favor (including written documents and statements from the company's own officers), I believe I would have won if I had had the needed strength and funds to keep fighting in the court system for the additional years that may have been required. However, I had not known what could happen by being tied up in the "justice" system, and over six years of my life had already been consumed in this legal battle. Time was on the company's side to drag it out even longer.

Earth Time Is Too Precious to Hold Grudges

Gratefully though, through Roger's skilled efforts, facts that were previously unknown to me were discovered about what had actually been taking place concerning my breached contract and stalled litigation. Facts were uncovered about important meetings that were held, monies that were paid, and agreements that had been made without my knowledge with adverse effects for my business interests. I do not believe this information would have been otherwise revealed.

Thereafter, hints began to surface that a settlement offer for several million dollars was going to be coming to me. Subsequently, though, everything seemed to stop; we heard nothing from those involved or from the court for some time. Then there was a devastating surprise ruling from the court which all of my attorneys saw as unfair and not consistent with the evidence that had been presented. It could have required months or even years of extended litigation to overcome.

The stress I had experienced dealing with this company and its spinoffs was almost unbearable. I had come to a point of depletion physically, financially, and emotionally. I was weak and on oxygen and having difficulty breathing. I realized that I had to close those painful chapters of my life, take my losses, forgive, forget, *let go*, and withdraw from the legal battle. I knew it would cost my life to continue this fight any longer, and I didn't believe that was what God wanted me to do.

Then, another surprise, but this time a pleasant one—an *unrequired* settlement offer was made which would almost take care of the high legal expenses I had accumulated over six years. With adjustments from my attorneys on their fees and expenses, the settlement covered their costs of this legal battle. My prayers had not been answered as I had hoped, but I knew what truly mattered was to go on with my life the best I could.

Drawing on the knowledge I gained when I was on the Other Side, I was extremely grateful to get through that very difficult period of time without being embittered. My prayers were answered with a peaceful feeling and with the assurance of rewards awaiting me on the Other Side instead of "justice" or "victory" or material blessings here. As I continued to pray, my sorrow was swallowed up in the God-given inner peace that is available to all. I knew within my heart that I had passed a *big test* because I did not have any bad feelings toward those who had hurt me with their callous actions.

At that time, I saw things in the eternal perspective, and I felt sorrow for how much they were hurting themselves and their posterity (by their bad example) when they face the consequences of their actions on the Other Side. I knew that God does not answer prayers by taking away others' free agency, and I couldn't blame God for the wrong choices others had made.

Because I knew I was exchanging my short allotment of time on Earth for whatever I did that day, I was striving to look more carefully at my priorities. Time on Earth is too short to remain angry or hold grudges against anyone; it is precious and limited when compared to the forever of eternity.

Thoughts Are Powerful

Each hour of the day, I know that I make choices which include deliberately taking control of my thinking or allowing other forces to sway, dictate, or manipulate my thoughts and attitudes. I know that attitudes and desires are formed as a direct result of thoughts held daily in my mind, which then determine what I will accomplish during my life on Earth.

Thoughts are powerful and too valuable to waste!

CHAPTER 42

Finding Hidden Benefits Reaps Rewards

Music in the Lunchroom

Several years ago, I became aware of a business owned by a husband and wife team. They badly needed financial backing; they were on the brink of folding a business I believed had great potential. At a meeting one evening, they were discussing the way the business would be set up after they moved to a new location. The wife was bubbling with ideas; she wanted the employees to have half a day off each week to play golf. She also wanted them to have a lunchroom where classical music would play continually and elevate them to new levels of productivity.

Her husband wanted to have western music played in the lunchroom, and he emphatically made his viewpoint known. The debate was on. Voices began to rise. The couple was getting very angry over the type of music to be played in the lunchroom of a building that hadn't even been rented yet. The lunchroom never did materialize, nor did a system on which to play any music.

A Better Perspective

Now, whenever I find myself beginning to fuss over differing points of view, I pause, take a deep breath and think, "Is this argument about music in the lunchroom?" Sometimes I laugh until tears roll down my cheeks as I stand back and see things from a better perspective.

It's amazing that people often get so involved in arguments that they could actually, physically hurt each other over something similar to "music in the lunchroom." This experience reinforced the lessons I learned on the Other Side about the futility of arguing. I find it much easier now to let others express their opinions without contradicting them. It's not up to me to challenge others' opinions and try to get them to see things my way. And

I feel free from the need to defend my position—it's easier to compassionately listen and *"let it go"* if we disagree.

Deadly Notions or Heavenly Rewards

On the Other Side, I became aware that there are many ways to handle problems in life. Running from them, though, and using drugs or drinking alcohol only makes them worse. Drugs and alcohol affect the chemicals in the brain and ultimately add to feeling depressed and overwhelmed—and can seriously damage health. They impair judgment and the ability to make decisions; problems of those who use them increase and compound.

Drugs, alcohol, and negative thoughts can insidiously steal life because, under their influence, people are more apt to act impulsively on the false and deadly notion that suicide is a glamorous, or acceptable way of escaping unwanted challenges—I was clearly shown that *it is not!*

Earth Time Is to Gather Good Deeds and Develop Good Character Traits

Life presents problems—working on them rather than hiding from them helps us find solutions. *Ignoring problems or blaming others does not solve them; facing them head on, praying for strength and guidance to solve them and the wisdom to find their hidden benefits, reaps great rewards.*

Others' Near-Death Experiences

On the Other Side I had questioned, "What about those who died, found a beautiful, peaceful place, and came back to Earth life again? Will they find that peace next time?" The answer was given me that it depends upon the intent of their hearts and their actions as it does for all of us. My understanding was reinforced with the knowledge that *we are required to endure whatever happens to us to the end of our lives.*

However, as well as I know this, there are times when I find certain unwanted, familiar feelings starting to return, and I have to replace them with thoughts I know will help to create the actions and results I really want. Knowing that if I let my mind dwell on upsetting, unhappy thoughts, I will again attract "bad-habit thinking," I stop those thoughts by remembering what I experienced on the Other Side. The principles I learned there help me make it through difficult situations.

157

CHAPTER 43

Life—Worth Living and Celebrating

When my perspective is clear, I gladly accept life's challenges and the size of my body. Whether I am slender or not is no longer a big issue for me. Before my near-death experience, I had been anorexic and bulimic. I had mistakenly thought that being "thin" was critically important to being happy.

However, on the Other Side, it was revealed to me and I was given knowledge and truth about the importance of having good health and that the popular desire to be thin is only a fad of present-day fashion.

Also, on the Other Side, I learned that anorexia, bulimia, or eating "junk food" can cause pain, stress, and extreme anxiety. It can kill us. How we treat our bodies can greatly determine the quality and length of our lives. The choices we make, the kinds and amounts of foods and water we eat and drink daily are definitely linked to how we think and feel.

I also learned that we need proper nourishment for body, mind, and spirit—they are absolutely intertwined. I was shown that our choices have Earthly and spiritual consequences, which build or deplete our energy. *Our bodies are gifts from God, and must last us a lifetime.*

Learning more about the natural health field has been fascinating, and implementing the knowledge is a day-today challenge. When I nourish my mind, body, and spirit, and depend on God's timing, I have discovered profound whisperings of the Spirit and reaped miracles.

As I write this, I am reminded of a message I put on a wall plaque. It is from the poem "Salutation to the Dawn," author unknown. I adapted and added to this saying, and sometimes I give it out at speaking engagements:

Yesterday is already a dream, tomorrow is only a vision; but today, WELL LIVED, makes every yesterday a dream of happiness, and tomorrow a vision of hope.
Celebrate Life. This Is Not a Dress Rehearsal!

The Need for Help Rather than Advice

Before my near-death experience in 1983, I had tried many different things through the years to help myself, but feelings of depression and thoughts of suicide continued to creep into my mind. Their luring appeal was based on false notions of escaping from life's problems and gaining unearned peace.

Friends and family offered advice such as, "Get hold of yourself," and phrases like, "Pull yourself together! How can you be blue when you have so many blessings?" and "Snap out of it!" When I was depressed to the point of considering suicide and I would hear, "Think of your family," it only made me feel more suicidal because I wrongly felt they were selfish to ask me to live when I wanted to die.

I would caution those approached by people voicing thoughts of suicide. Statements that may seem like good advice are usually not well received by someone feeling downhearted and overwhelmed. "Get hold of yourself" type of comments do not help but add to their feelings of hopelessness, inadequacy, and can make them feel worse and even push them deeper into depression.

If it were always possible for people feeling extremely depressed to pull themselves together and get on with their lives, there would be few people with depression. It's important to realize when people feel depressed for an extended period of time, they may no longer be able to pull their mood up by themselves. They need help!

There are ways to help the suicidal person realize his or her own life's value: *All involved need to seek help.*

Take Control and Fight for Life

If you are the one feeling depressed, listen to your feelings and the whisperings of the Spirit. *Seek help actively!* Ask for it. Don't be put off. Go to a doctor, a religious leader, a counselor. *Fight for life. Pray and pray again!* We are each responsible for our own happiness. Taking control of our thoughts, feelings, attitudes, and consequently our lives often means seeking out the best resources we can find to help us solve our particular problems. I have discovered that I must be a detective searching out ideas and resources to make life as full as I can for myself in caring for my mind, body, and spirit. I know that I must be aware of my moods and continually remind myself of my true purpose for living and of the true, lasting peace of mind to be found in right thinking.

I feel I must warn as many people as possible, any who will listen to what I discovered: *We are our own judges!* When we get to the Other Side too soon and realize what we gave up and the sorrow or pain we caused others, we may experience an emotional torture of our own making that is true agony.

The Great Benefits of Hanging On

There are times in life when you may be faced with the choice of giving up on life or going on. Please hear my message. *Life is worth living!*

Choosing otherwise can steal away great joys. It is not a chance worth taking. I learned that life offers rich opportunities even in seeming defeats. Glorious rewards can be earned and enjoyed in this life, and *especially* on the Other Side, with right thoughts, actions, and kind deeds.

Life-Threatening Myths

Circumstances are constantly changing—often for the better. At least during Earth life, we can still repent, find solutions, and grow wiser. *Death is so final.* Suicidal thoughts are false, futile attempts to escape from problems, rather than solve them. They short-circuit thinking and add to problems and feelings of depression. Suicidal thoughts always contain *life-threatening myths!*

Suicidal thoughts actually stopped me from finding solutions.

When I was on the Other Side, the anguish from my wrong actions created an unquenchable burning and searing of my conscience. It was agonizing to realize I had lost great rewards of happiness as a result of my choices when enduring and hanging on a little longer could have brought me the rewards of eternal victory with my family and loved ones.

I feel that it is important to again repeat that only God knows the full answers to questions regarding those who commit suicide and only He can administer a fair judgment and decide the degree of each person's accountability. However, even though individuals may feel depressed and miserable in life, they *may* feel enormously worse on the Other Side if they end their lives.

One of God's Greatest Gifts

During my near-death experience, I learned that life is one of God's greatest gifts to each of us. To throw it away by committing suicide is possibly one of the worst acts one can commit—it is offensive and disrespectful to Him. Suicide is a tragedy for all concerned.

Also, I learned that when a person has sincerely tried to meet their challenges and it is their time to die, they can pass on to a welcoming home from those who love them on the Other Side and enjoy the fruits of their labors on Earth. He or she can look forward to the harvest of good deeds and good attitudes by having endured well to the end. Such individuals will be met by heavenly family, friends, angels, and God with mutual rejoicing over Earthly achievements.

CHAPTER 44

Highlights from Heaven: an Overview

My experience was the most realistic event of my life. While I was on the Other Side all of my senses were expanded beyond anything possible in mortal life. By comparison, Earth life is the dream world. Realism is only found on the Other Side.

Taking just one example, that of knowledge—never during Earth life could my mind have grasped what it did there. It was as if I were drinking from some vast pool of forgotten wisdom. Information poured into me the instant I formulated a question. And much of what I knew over there seemed to come from within me, as if from a dormant pool that had suddenly become energized in this different sphere.

A Sphere of Love

It was a different sphere—one in which knowledge was readily available to the earnest seeker and one in which the concept of time is meaningless. The past, present, and future seemed accessible on demand. And the place was permeated with love—love that rises to emotional heights undreamed of in Earthly terms.

A Great Retirement Fund in Heaven

Another Great Truth that I learned while I was on the Other Side is that enduring well while making it through problems during Earth life will bring such great satisfaction and peace of mind over there that it defies description. It is like discovering that there is a *great retirement fund in heaven* which is built by overcoming problems during Earth life with loving, forgiving, and charitable attitudes and actions. Such actions create heavenly rewards that include lasting, eternal peace and joy.

What I saw was not pleasant, and added to the realism of the experience. Those who had committed suicide, for example, I saw that they were pitifully distraught people who had somehow broken a premortal promise to make the most of their lives. Their agony of missed opportunity was clearly evident; I shared some of their feelings because I had willed myself to die.

Life's events, good and bad, were put into an eternal perspective that finally made sense to me. Never, with the dim Earthly understanding I had before my experience, could I have fathomed the meaning and purposes of life as I did there. I came to understand that Earthly life is a gift precious beyond belief.

Another Chance

My return to life was a wondrous, welcome reprieve. My choice to return was driven by my desire to remedy my approach to life and its problems. With my new understanding of what I could have been, life, with all of its trials and challenges, became an exciting adventure with almost limitless opportunities. If I successfully dealt with those opportunities, then a boundless future awaited me—an expansive future, in a marvelous, glorious sphere, limited only by my own thoughts and actions.

It is difficult to put into words what I saw and felt on the Other Side. The anguish, the peace, the light, the scenes, the sounds, the expanded feelings and increased knowledge were magnificent, yet familiar. It eventually struck me that everything there was as it ought to be, a considerably different and marvelously strange world, not a replica of Earth-life's sphere.

Healing Defies Medical Wisdom

Other events after my return gave further evidence of the reality of my experience. The healing I enjoyed after my horribly debilitating illness, although not complete, was sufficient to allow me to realize my new-found life's mission. This healing defied most medical wisdom of the time. My recognition of the devastation created by my infected tooth was unexplainable by the best medical help I could get at the time. Yet the tooth's removal proved the efficacy of my Other Side's vision.

CHAPTER 45

Warning Signs Overlooked

At this point, in 1988, my muscle weakness persisted. I had problems walking and had to wear a neck brace to hold my head up, plus an ankle brace. Previously, I had been making excuses, saying, "I just need to exercise more," or "I've been under a lot of stress."

I started having muscle cramps and muscle twitching. The twitching worsened day by day. I felt like I had something bouncing around under my skin. I later learned these were called fasciculations.

Other symptoms that I had for the past couple of years, such as difficulty swallowing and breathing, as well as dropping things, became more pronounced and serious. I began to severely choke on my own saliva. My eyelids were badly drooping. To make matters worse, I had lost most of my voice. People had difficulty understanding me and I was embarrassed and reluctant to speak and have conversations.

CHAPTER 46

ALS Diagnosis

Although I was frightened and tried to deny these symptoms, I knew I needed to find out what was wrong. In May of 1988, I sought the help of Dr. Willem Khoe, a renowned medical doctor who also practiced homeopathy, acupuncture and traditional Chinese medicine in Las Vegas, Nevada.

He diagnosed me with myasthenia gravis (MG), but told me that some of my symptoms were not consistent with it, and that I also had ALS, amyotrophic lateral sclerosis, or Lou Gehrig's disease. Because of my problems breathing, he immediately gave me a prescription to be on oxygen.

The myasthenia gravis (MG) had masked many of my ALS symptoms. Some of the symptoms are similar, but ALS has additional symptoms that are totally different. As an example, muscles may weaken, but do not atrophy with MG, as they do with ALS.

Dr. Khoe was the first medical professional to diagnose me with ALS. At the time, I had no idea what it was. Even though MG is also a potentially life-threatening disease, and I still have to take medication for it regularly, he said that he could only focus on the ALS.

Despite my doubts, I trusted Dr. Khoe and agreed to the weekly treatments. He ordered the remedies and we started the treatments the following week.

When I went home, I researched ALS and found there were about 5,000 new cases per year in the United States, and about 220,000 worldwide. I became extremely frightened. Could Dr. Khoe possibly be wrong?

This disease appeared to be fatal, and have no cure. I was only in my fifties. I thought to myself, "Is this why I went to the 'Other Side', so I could die from ALS?"

Deciding I wanted a second opinion, I went to a very knowledgeable and experienced Naturopathic Physician. He performed various tests and also concluded that I had ALS.

Even though I had all these scary symptoms, doubts still plagued my mind. I just could not accept that I had this paralyzing, fatal disease. In order to be sure that my diagnosis was correct, in June of 1988 I sought out a third doctor. This one was a neurologist who had experience with ALS at a clinic in Salt Lake City, Utah.

He confirmed the diagnosis, and said, "You're doing very well for the stage you're in. Stick out your tongue and you will see that you cannot hold it still. You should make it to Thanksgiving."

As I stuck out my quivering tongue, I realized he was right. I had been in total denial. Thanksgiving was a mere five months away. I was 54 years old.

Not knowing what else to do, I began going to ALS support groups. The first one I attended was in Utah. The message was clear: "Do whatever you want, because you're going to die anyway. It doesn't matter what you think or what doctor you go to, because nothing can be done."

During a trip to southern California, I found another support group. Again, the talk was negative: "You're going to die, so just accept it." I thought, "No wonder people lost hope of recovering from this disease."

The one thing I did know was that if I were going to get better, it would not be by being around people who think like *this!*

CHAPTER 47

An Answer to Prayers

Having been to the Other Side, I knew there was hope for a miracle.

When I had previously gone to Dr. Khoe, he told me about a treatment from Germany for ALS. He said that a remarkable number of the people who were given a special homeopathic remedy recovered. Unfortunately, Dr. Khoe passed away in 1992, and I have not yet been able to find an equivalent homeopathic remedy.

In America, there were no known survivors that I knew about. Years later, I found out there actually was an ALS survivor. Her name is Evy McDonald. Dr. Khoe had told me he could not make any promises, but at this point, I felt I had nothing to lose, and that's why I decided to go ahead with the treatment.

The homeopathic remedy was mixed with my own blood, and then injected into specific acupuncture points. I agreed to try a course of one shot a week for ten weeks, even though I had to travel about 900 miles round trip to Las Vegas each time I received a treatment. My mother was kind enough to accompany me. It made the long trips go by faster.

During one of my early visits to Dr. Khoe in Las Vegas, I attended an ALS support group there. In Utah and California, neurologists ran the meetings, documented each person's worsening conditions, cut off anyone who had a positive story to share and instead told patients what to expect as the disease progressed towards death.

In Nevada, it was a very different experience. The ALS patients complained that they rarely got to see a neurologist. The meetings were conducted by a social worker.

What surprised me as an observer was that the ALS patients in the Nevada group seemed to be living years longer than either the Utah or the California group. In the Nevada group, all of them *walked* by themselves into the meeting even though, on average, it was years longer since their diagnosis than either of the other two groups, most of whom were already in wheelchairs or used scooters.

To this day, I have no doubt that it was because there was no neurologist telling them how soon they were going to die. In addition, instead of listening to patients list their worsening conditions to the neurologist, the Nevada ALS patients shared more of what they were doing that gave them motivation to live.

At this point, I decided not to attend ALS support groups anymore. There was nothing there that was going to help me. In fact, I felt it was discouraging.

Instead, I focused on getting well and not allowing any negative thoughts to enter my mind.

I continued the homeopathic treatment as well as prayer, maintaining a relentlessly positive mental attitude and consistently listening to *sleep learning* and meditating daily.

During treatment, Dr Khoe advised me to stop consuming meat products due to the hormones and antibiotics the animals were given. At the time, I did not believe that what I ate made much difference, so after one treatment I went right out to the nearest fast-food place and had a huge double cheeseburger!

Not long after this incident, driving home with my mom from Las Vegas, we parked our RV at a truck stop next to a big field. The following morning, I awoke to loud mooing and a terrible odor coming from a huge cattle truck parked right next to us—despite *all* of the many other open spaces where he could have parked. The cows were staring straight at me, accusingly, through the holes and bars of their mobile prison.

At that moment I remembered my doctor's advice about not eating meat, and decided to give it up then and there during the treatments. Those poor cows really got my attention! To me, this was a clear message from God.

I improved my diet, continued to pray, and listened to my recorded positive affirmations during the day and *sleep learning* at night. These recordings helped reduce the tremendous stress I was under. I knew it was important to stay positive.

Still, I had doubts. It was becoming harder and harder to walk. My choking got so bad I was embarrassed to eat in public. I even thought I might die from choking before the ALS had a chance to kill me.

My voice deteriorated to the point that I knew if it got much worse I would need something to communicate with others, so I looked for a voice board so people could point to a word or letter and I could acknowledge yes or no by blinking my eyes.

Around this time my lawsuit was still in progress, but my doctors sent notes to the court that because of my condition after my ALS diagnosis I was unable to withstand the stress of depositions or testimony.

Had I been forced to testify at this time, I was certain the stress would have killed me. (Later, when my deposition was taken, it lasted *many* very stressful days.)

After the 10 weeks of homeopathic treatments, and 9000 miles of driving, I saw only mild improvements. I certainly didn't feel cured by the end of it. What now? If the remedy was going to work, the ALS should have been on the way out by now.

Then Dr. Khoe went on vacation, I missed my homeopathic injection that week and we both noticed I didn't do as well without it. After talking with him, he agreed to let me have the shots for a few more weeks.

Meanwhile, I kept on praying, but with even greater frequency and intensity. I also continued to listen to and mentally recite positive affirmations throughout the day so that I could better control my thoughts, feelings and actions.

After praying with a close friend and believer, we were left with the strong conviction that, in this particular case, it was my choice whether I would live or die. I was praying to live and doing my best to make it so. In addition, I prepared myself spiritually in case God had other plans for me.

In the prayer, I was also told if I decided to live, God was going to bless my voice. For someone in my compromised physical condition who lost their voice, this seemed hard to believe. Still, I prayed that it was true.

One day, a few days after receiving my last shot of the homeopathic remedy, during a sincere heartfelt prayer, I felt something change.

I remember it was as if a light gray smoke had lifted up off me.

A short while later my husband stated that "something was different" about me, and I seemed better. I sensed it too. I felt stronger and the choking stopped.

Immediately, I felt improvement in many ways, and in the coming weeks I noticed my muscle wasting stopped its progression.

My doctor gave me some tests. Afterwards, he declared that my ALS was gone.

It was a miracle.

My energy and strength quickly returned to normal.

The choking episodes and muscle twitching completely stopped.

After more time, my voice fully recovered, and even now at almost 90 years old, I am often mistaken on the phone for a much younger person.

CHAPTER 48

A Letter from Dr. Logan

While writing this book, I had a conversation with Dr. Logan, who was one of my three doctors during my ALS recovery. I am including his letter here as part of my story.

February 12, 2021

To Whom It May Concern:

Joyce has been a patient of mine over many years. I am unable to find her original file, but it was around the early 1980s when I first saw her. In the later part of the 1980s, having treated her before she was ill, I became aware of changes in her complaints, symptoms, and physical condition. She had weakness, muscle atrophy, choking problems, and loss of most of her voice. She was also on oxygen because of her breathing problems. I did some tests and it appeared she had ALS.

Dr. Willem Khoe, MD, in Las Vegas also diagnosed ALS for Joyce. I have met him and knew that he had used some alternative medical techniques that worked well for her. My findings and additional neurologists Joyce had seen were consistent with Dr. Khoe's diagnoses that she was in an advanced stage of ALS.

I saw Joyce soon after she completed her treatments with Dr. Khoe and she had none of her former ALS complaints or symptoms.

To this day, even at almost 90 years, she has the voice of a much younger person and leads an extremely active life. She is an author of several books, speaker, founder and president of Stress and Grief Relief, Inc., a non-profit organization for suicide prevention, including a life-saving hotline. Her website is www.hopedr.org.

This letter is to verify my personal knowledge of over thirty years of Joyce Brown's medical history, including her battle with ALS in 1988. I trust this will help with the direction of Joyce's present research into understanding this disease and the giving of hope to those who are searching for answers.

Sincerely yours,

Cordell E. Logan, Ph.D., ND.

CHAPTER 49

The ALS Reversal Recipe that Worked for Me

People often ask me what things I did to reverse ALS, and what I do now if I have health problems. I believe that the miraculous healing of my ALS in 1988 was a combination of the following:

1. Prayer and a sincere personal relationship with God
2. Removal of all of the amalgam fillings (i.e. mercury and silver) from my teeth
3. Skilled homeopathy and acupuncture
4. A major change of diet, including striving to eat organic, giving up non-grass-fed meat, and drinking adequate amounts of filtered water.
5. *Belief* that I could heal, which was profoundly influenced by my near-death experience
6. Listening to my *sleep learning* recordings *Whispers for Life & Prosperity*, and *Whispers for Miraculous Results* (see image below), which gave me a positive attitude towards life and increased my own body's ability to heal, and
7. A specialized, personalized meditation using the CD of *Whispers for Miraculous Results*.

As a result of decades of study and experience, I have found there are great health benefits from these additional practices:

1. A doctor that can administer an intravenous (IV) of vitamins and minerals, especially one that is high in Vitamin C and Glutathione.
2. A physician trained to use ozone therapy that increases the oxygen in the blood in order to build the immune system.
3. Deep breathing of pure, clean air.
4. Increase the body's healing energy, which is affected by what we eat, drink, and think, including prayer, but also how we are impacted by the energy in our environment, including how well we manage stress.

This is my personal basic recipe that I have recommended. However, there is additional information that is helping others with reversals at: HealingALS.org.

CHAPTER 50

A Miraculous Healing

Though three doctors had diagnosed me, and the symptoms are easily found on the internet, I have always been reluctant to talk about having had ALS, let alone the story of my miraculous recovery—that is, until now, when numerous others are telling about their ALS reversals.

When I wrote my book, *God's Heavenly Answers*, I only referred to my ALS as the broader group of diseases known as *Muscular Dystrophy*. At the time, no one else I knew of was talking about healing ALS, and I didn't want to be the first, nor did I want that to become the focus of my book.

One day in September of 2014, Patricia Tamowski called from New York and told me that she and her husband, Scott Douglas, were professional filmmakers. They were interviewing people who had ALS reversals and wanted to hear my story of recovery.

After asking her if I was the first one she had found, and learning I was the tenth, I agreed to share my personal experience. Patricia and Scott found out about me after tracking down an acquaintance of mine, a male in his forties who was also healed of ALS.

There was no way of knowing at the time what a great relationship would develop between us. In the beginning, I still found it very difficult to talk about. But shortly after Patricia contacted me, I started to open up. I gave Patricia permission to share my number with people who had ALS, and wanted to call and ask me questions, but I still felt slightly uncomfortable.

One day while sitting at the table in the kitchen thinking about not wanting to talk about my ALS experience, I suddenly heard a distinct voice say,

"I helped you!"

Instantly, a feeling swept over my whole body; I felt a deep sense of gratitude for being healed of ALS. I immediately felt a new desire to share my experience, and what I believe could help others, with the hope and possibility that they too could have a miraculous healing. I now had a new desire, and a deeper awareness of the importance of sharing my story with people who have ALS.

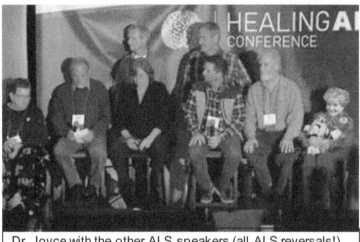

Dr. Joyce with the other ALS speakers (all ALS reversals!)

CHAPTER 51

Sharing My ALS Story

Over the next few years Patricia and Scott came to my home to film, take pictures, and interview me about the various life-and-death adventures and miracles of my life. They even took a video of me dancing the twist with Scott (see photo below) showing how I had no after-effects from the ALS. This was also the time I was elated to see both Patricia and Scott at my public speaking competition where I was the International Toastmasters award-winning contestant for Southern Utah in 2018 at age 84. The title of my speech was, "Life is Worth Living." Meanwhile, they continued to gather information, and conduct interviews, many of which are published on their YouTube channel Healing Advocates.

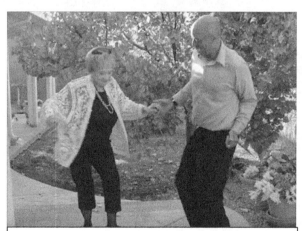

Dr. Joyce dancing "The Twist" with Scott Douglas.

Patricia and Scott found other people who had healed from ALS, as well as those who were in different stages of the disease who needed hope and help. During their research they became acquainted with Richard Bedlack, M.D., Ph.D., Director of Duke University's ALS Clinic. As part of his research at Duke, Dr. Bedlack tracks and documents ALS reversals and, at present, has *confirmed* approximately 50 ALS reversals around the world. If you are interested in learning more about ALS reversals, I highly recommend you get in touch with Patricia and Scott who are currently learning about even more ALS reversals.

Since I started writing this book, I have learned of another 12 ALS reversals attributed to prayer, as well as 5 others attributed to homeopathy. This is exciting news and we are expecting to hear of many additional ALS reversals soon.

When Dr. Bedlack's colleague contacted me, requesting information about my medical history and recovery from ALS and having myasthenia gravis (MG), I was interested to learn from him that, even though it is rare, many of the ALS cases that he was studying also had MG.

After considerable organizing, preparation and pre-work, Patricia and Scott hosted the world's first ever Healing ALS Conference from the 18th to the 20th of October 2019 (www.HealingALSConference.org).

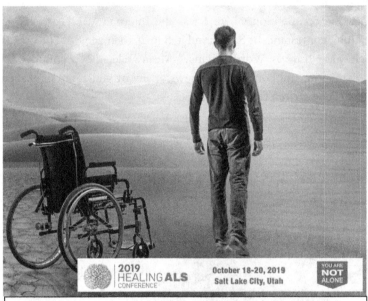

2019 HEALING ALS CONFERENCE   October 18-20, 2019 Salt Lake City, Utah   YOU ARE NOT ALONE

The 2019 Healing ALS Conference graphic, designed by Steve Arscott, a beloved member of the ALS community (diagnosed in 2013).

Held at the Radisson Hotel in Downtown Salt Lake City, the event was a spectacular success. Nearly 300 people attended the conference from over 10 different countries. The conference was also live-streamed to more than 25 nations around the world, with nearly 1,000 people tuning in.

It was a great privilege to be one of eight speakers with a complete reversal of ALS at the conference, and to share my life story of how I was miraculously healed in 1988. My slide presentation included pictures from my near-death experience, and my book, *God's Heavenly Answers*, as well as my *sleep learning* recordings with their powerful positive affirmations, *Whispers for Miraculous Results*. As I pointed out in my speech, along with the steps I outlined earlier, I believe the recordings were a tremendously important part of my healing.

Knowing that the audience was filled with people who had ALS, as well as their caregivers, family, and friends, my heart was so touched that, as I shared my story, I could not hold back my tears.

I couldn't see them; however, it was as if I could personally feel their heartaches and challenges. Many were in power chairs, and differing stages of ALS. There was even one wife pushing her husband in a wheeled gurney, because he was too advanced with ALS to be able to sit up.

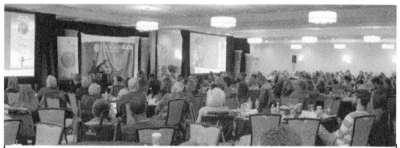

The audience from the Healing ALS Conference, including 300 in-person attendees and live-streamed to another 3,000 people in 30 countries around the world. Dr. Joyce is seated on stage speaking about her complete reversal from ALS back in 1988.

As the first Healing ALS conference, it was the only place in the world where there was hope and healing information available, as well as selected experts and top doctors who were there to share valuable information about ALS. I felt very grateful to have been healed of ALS in 1988, and I was honored to be there to share my story and offer hope that others can receive miracles too.

Since that conference, phone calls, letters and emails have been coming in continuously from people all over the world, who are advancing toward ALS reversal after what they learned. For more information about the conference and priceless information from leading experts in the field about health and healing, go to their website www.HealingALS.org.

We are also receiving letters and emails from people sharing their own success stories and miraculous results from using our unique coping techniques, *sleep learning* and other life-changing, life-saving information.

To learn more about the methods I personally used, go to our website www.HopeDr.org. You will also find life-changing books, articles, positive, stress relieving affirmations, recordings that help you learn while you sleep, meditations and so much more. Additionally, you will find information about how to have hope, reap miracles, and find relief from stress, depression and grief.

Still today, knowing that people need help and answers *now*, I feel a great urgency to make my books and recordings available as quickly as possible.

CHAPTER 52

Creating Miraculous Results

Due to the fact that I have serious spinal issues, I only have so much time each day before I need to lie down. In addition to having visual impairment, these challenges make whatever miraculous results I'm striving for more complicated and time consuming.

I wholeheartedly believe that many different ailments I've recovered from and the calamities I've conquered over the years were influenced by my positive, purposeful, mentally programmed *belief* that I *would* recover, and furthermore, that I had not yet finished my real purpose for living.

Since my near-death experience, and personally knowing to whom I am praying, my prayers are now much deeper, more like a two-way conversation, as I listen for whisperings of the Spirit.

Whenever I think about what I might have done differently, looking back on my life and my ordeal with ALS, I wish I had picked up on and paid attention to my symptoms sooner—warning signs which had been going on far longer than I realized. However, considering all the stress I was under with the lawsuit, the symptoms seemed insignificant compared to everything else that was happening.

I now encourage others to take quick action when they sense that something is not right with their health, but also to have courage, faith, pray, and listen for promptings and direction from above.

Heavenly whisperings and interventions work differently for different people, although listening is always key. During my near-death experience, I received guidance about my infected gold-crowned tooth with its silver fillings containing mercury.

Some people receive information and promptings with soft whisperings of the Spirit during prayers, reading scriptures, through dreams or simply by talking with others, or even by consulting with various specialists.

I should have been more in-tune with my own health, gone to see a specialist sooner, and changed my diet. Even now, when I stray too far from eating the right foods, I pay for it with health challenges, and have to get myself back in line.

I have found, in both my personal and professional experience, that many people who choose not to rely solely on the traditional medical establishment, tend to live healthier and longer lives.

While the conventional medical community is needed for many injuries and illnesses, looking outside of it allowed me to find the help that ultimately healed me.

Again, I'd like to emphasize the specific areas that I focused on, and have found most helpful for hope and healing, including the following: prayer, finding a purpose for living, homeopathy, along with acupuncture, holistic dentistry and getting amalgam fillings removed and replaced properly, listening to positive affirmations while you sleep, positive thinking and overall changing my attitude towards life, stress relief, with meditation, a healthy diet, and proper rest and exercise. Different things work for different people and their particular conditions, these are the main things that worked for me.

Often, I am asked to share the 2 or 3 most important factors on this list, however in my mind, all these suggestions rank number one.

My beliefs are based on my education and experience as a Naturopathic Medical Doctor (N.M.D.), working with renowned medical experts and scientists, as well as my personal knowledge with my own health and other people I have helped.

Holistic medicine takes work and research. Carrying out various protocols can be intense. At times working with a holistic MD and a nutritional specialist is invaluable. It is worth it though, for all the extra years of having loved ones in our lives, and the increased health and quality of life during those years.

If you go to a doctor or health specialist you aren't comfortable with, keep searching for a practitioner who shares your outlook, and helps you achieve the best possible results. Every doctor has his or her own training and perspective.

In addition, based on my observations, support groups which permit participants to share positive experiences and support one another seem to have better outcomes.

In 1988, the only option I knew about was to attend a group which focused on death, dying, and decline. Our present group, *Healing ALS,* with Patricia and Scott, inspires, encourages, and enlightens with a focus on hope and healing as well as sharing stories of successful ALS reversals.

For additional facts and information, as well as the most recent accounts, visit their website www.HealingALS.org.

The site is a storehouse of wisdom, knowledge and stories of peoples' improvements and ALS reversals, including my own account (see Dr. Joyce Brown's ALS Reversal Story Part 1, and Dr. Joyce Brown Q&A Part 2). Also, on You Tube are several videos under Dr. Joyce Brown Suicide Prevention. Other videos may be found on the website HopeDr.org as you browse the menu or use our search tool.

When asked why I was permitted to have another chance to live after my near-death experience, and why I didn't die from ALS when so many other good and deserving people have lost their lives, I can only say that I don't know.

Perhaps, at that time, I had not yet fulfilled my purpose here on Earth. We do not always know what God's plans are for each of us. If someone has done everything they can possibly do for their own health, if they are treating others with kindness and forgiveness, and if they are living the best they can each day, then it makes sense to make peace with their family and themselves, make the most of each moment, and trust God's will.

Even with sincere and repeated prayers, answers do not always come quickly or easily. Our timing and God's timing are not always the same. Sometimes it takes weeks, months, or even years of prayers to get the answer or miracle we seek.

When a miracle is needed, the road can be long and difficult before we feel we are connected and have a direct line to heaven.

Yet, often when we least expect it, we can receive a miraculous answer to our prayers directly from God. I know this firsthand, and if it happened for me, *I know it can happen for anyone.*

CHAPTER 53

After ALS

After my recovery from ALS, I still had the lawsuit to contend with, which required an enormous amount of my attention. The court case dragged on with tremendous pressure from all of their attorneys.

After all that I had been going through, other health problems surfaced, and the stress was causing my myasthenia gravis (MG) symptoms to worsen.

I realized I needed to move on from a battle that was threatening my health and life.

To improve my health, and my life, I decided to forgo compensation for my losses, and in 1992, I accepted a settlement that barely covered the legal fees.

The worst part was the heartbreak of knowing that the 500 tons per day of solid waste garbage, *including plastic bags, bottles, and straws*, was no longer going to be converted to energy in my plant. Instead, it would be dumped into the landfill. Because of tradition and convenience, and because what is right and good does not always prevail, this process of putting most of the waste into landfills, versus converting it to energy, continues in most areas to this day.

It really hurt to leave behind that part of my life working in the alternative energy and hazardous waste fields. It was very depressing to know that there are solutions for pollution control and energy shortages that are not being implemented.

With the court case lasting six years, I felt overwhelmed and just wanted to become a different person. After all of those years of being in court with our lawsuit, so many financial losses, and dealing with attorney's, I felt extremely victimized.

When they breached the contract, laid off employees and left my project in about May of 1986, I quickly realized I needed to change fields and begin a whole new way of life.

No longer being able to help cities or counties, I decided I would focus on helping individuals with their spiritual, mental, and health issues. I realized this would require new intense studies, spiritual guidance, and miracles. I became deeply and actively engrossed in learning about the vast field of holistic health.

After God answered my pleadings with another chance to live, as I promised Him, my soul's sincere desire was to help people so they will enjoy the Other Side when they get there.

The lawsuit itself, however, was also turning out to be a tremendous learning experience. Five and a half years into it, facing some seventeen different attorneys in court, I decided I wanted to learn more about the law. In fact, I developed a deep desire to know more about the legal world which surrounds us.

After making a few inquiries, an associate suggested I check with the University of West Los Angeles Law School for more information. I knew I didn't have the time, energy, or money to go to law school, but I wanted to learn more about the bigger picture, so I called and asked if they had any courses available that I could take to learn about the legal system. I was quite surprised when they told me of a 5-week "post graduate" program that they were about to launch as part of their Professional Advancement Series. They billed the series of concentrated lectures—covering everything from contracts, torts, and wills to legal research, judicial process, and criminal law—as a "mini law school," and which amounted to a condensed version of a legal education.

Determined to no longer feel victimized and uninformed, I immediately signed up for the program, commuting about 200 miles round-trip for each class. After all the travel and work, I was thrilled when I received the post-graduate certificate in June 1991 which, along with everything I learned, more than satisfied my quest for legal knowledge. Rather than being afraid of the law and tricky lawyers, I now felt like I was part of it. I also felt empowered to utilize the law should it ever become necessary. I remain a firm believer in the power of education as a solution to many of life's most stubborn problems.

What a contrast to when I was a little girl, only two weeks into the first grade. I still remember sitting on the bench outside the principal's office, determined I would never willingly go back to school. With this constant reluctance, and the belief that I didn't need schooling, I was consistently on the absentee list for several years. However, in high school, I quickly learned there were few jobs available for those without an adequate education. Now, finally, I became a sponge for learning.

Over time, I developed an unquenchable thirst for knowledge. Ultimately, God blessed me with the desire and ability to become proficient in multiple fields of science as related to personal health. Before long I became a Master Life Coach and a Certified National Health Practitioner. I also earned a certification in the Quantum Energy Field (QEF) as an International Biofeedback Therapist.

But the more I learned, the more I realized how much more there is to learn, and the more I wanted to continue learning. As I continued my education in psychology, I started taking a deeper interest in how people deal with trauma and stress. I eventually became a Board-Certified Expert in Traumatic Stress and, years later, a Certified Crisis Chaplain with the American Academy of Experts in Traumatic Stress.

Fortunately, the countless hours of training and study quickly started paying off for others. In fact, I remember being surprised and deeply gratified by the extent to which my training, particularly advanced holistic therapies, was helping people overcome both their physical and emotional ailments. I was amazed by the power of these tools, and I wondered why they were not more mainstream, a part of every clinical practice.

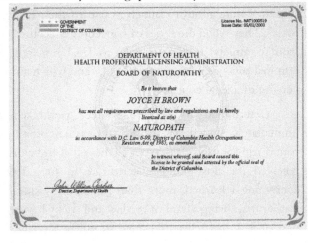

Ultimately, after working closely with several top medical doctors, experts who *were* open to advanced alternative treatments, I was invited to join various medical teams in private practice as an N.M.D., including Dr. José Calzada, who told me that he considered me "a fellow colleague." Dr.

Calzada, who has long been known for being on the cutting-edge of medicine, wanted me to join his clinic to offer these advanced holistic therapies to his patients. As honored as I was by his recognition and generous invitation, I felt my life purpose was taking me in a different direction. To this day, Dr. Calzada continues to lead the way with his advanced, holistic approach to medicine.

What I learned above all from this period of great learning and growth, was that there is a tremendous amount of wisdom and knowledge out there, well beyond what you find within the confines of each segmented field or discipline, including medicine. In other words, whether in business, psychology, medicine or law, the experts have only a fraction of all there is to know in their field, and the discipline itself is severely limited by accepted conventions, orthodoxies, and beliefs.

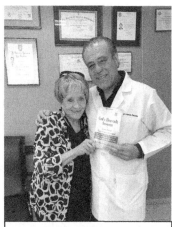

Dr. Joyce with Dr. José Calzada at his office.

I share all of this not to impress you, but to impress upon you that there is hope and possible answers for even the most difficult of life's questions, even when the doctors say that there is nothing else that can be done.

I share this to impress upon you the reality of all of the *unfound* knowledge in the world, and all the *possibilities* that may yet await you, well after you believe, as I did, that your life is nearing its end.

CHAPTER 54

Pathways to Being a Better Messenger

After hearing some great motivational speakers, I wanted to know more about how they developed such wonderful speaking skills. I soon learned they were members of the National Speakers Association (NSA). The NSA has regular meetings and classes, with a local chapter in most large cities.

In order to be a better messenger for God, I joined the NSA in 1987, and quickly found the meetings to be a thrilling change of pace.

I was exceptionally fortunate to get to know personally and learn directly from Cavett Robert, the man who founded the NSA back in 1973. I also met and became well acquainted with Dr. Norman Vincent Peale, the celebrated author of *The Power of Positive Thinking*. Furthermore, I got to know other great legends in the speaking world including Patricia Fripp, Art Berg, Kathy Loveless, and Jeanne Robertson. During this very exciting time, I learned that Australia was even more interested in self-help subjects than the United States. This idea really captured my attention.

I talked with Cavett Robert and Norman Vincent Peale about the possibility and opportunities for the three of us to make a trip to Australia. They thought it was a great idea and plans started falling into place. This is when I first created the expanded version of my *sleep learning* CDs, including *Whispers for Life and Prosperity*, *Whispers for Zest and Cheer for Peace of Mind*, and *Whispers of the Sea of Knowledge*.

However, due to the time-consuming requirements of the lawsuit, it turned out that I was not able to go with them as we had planned.

Over the years, I have often wondered how my life would have been different if I *had* been able to join them on that trip to Australia, helping individuals who wanted to change their lives for the better.

Instead, I studied and took courses and became a Naturopathic Medical Doctor (N.M.D.) with special training in both traditional and alternative medicine. Now looking back over my life, I can see that this was a much better path for my life's purpose. My life was filled with unexpected challenges.

On Father's Day 1998, my husband Earl was experiencing some minor chest pains. We decided to drive to the emergency room to have him checked out. They said that everything was okay, but that they would keep Earl overnight for evaluation. They insisted that I should go home. While driving on the freeway, I felt a soft, but distinct touch on my left shoulder. At the same time, I felt a wave come over my whole being, and I heard Earl's voice telling me that he was on the Other Side. Within less than a minute, I received a call from the hospital telling me to come back. Earl had passed away.

Rather than living only a few weeks, as the doctors said when his heart troubles were first diagnosed in 1984, Earl had lived actively for another 14 years, even with the multiple other serious medical issues he had, ultimately dying of accidental asphyxiation.

As shocked and grief-stricken as I was and as worried as I was about financial obligations and losing the house, I also felt a soft penetrating message from the Lord letting me know that it was Earl's time to come home.

Right after his death, I had an accident and I fell off a step ladder breaking both ankles.

Even though I was deeply grieving and in physical pain, I realized from my near-death experience that I needed to move forward, and make the best use of my own limited Earth time to get God's message out.

CHAPTER 55

Radio Talk Show Host Question That Changed My Life

One day in August of 1998, I happened to see a flyer that caught my interest. It was a special class for authors who wanted to be a guest speaker on radio talk shows to share their message.

The flyer seemed to come out of nowhere, and I thought to myself that this is just what I needed. The class was conducted by the renowned former prime-time talk show host, Joel D. Roberts.

I knew I needed this class. The class was once a week and was 75 miles away. Even though it was painfully difficult, I made the 150 mile round trip every Saturday for 5 weeks.

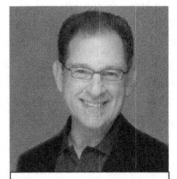

Prime-time talk show host Joel D. Roberts.

There were about 17 people wanting to promote their books in the class, each with various different religious beliefs; including Christian, Christian Scientist, Jewish, but also Atheists and Agnostics.

Knowing of their different beliefs, I felt overwhelmingly intimidated, and was reluctant to speak about my near-death experience and personal message from God.

Joel, the instructor, was sitting at a big round table with a practice microphone (which was not even plugged in). He gave instructions about how to be an interesting guest on a talk show. He even gave tips on how to handle a host when he or she asked questions that might put you in an uncomfortable position. For example, anticipating difficult questions and practicing answering them with confidence.

Knowing the differing beliefs that everyone else in the class had about God, each time my turn came I felt very intimidated and reluctant to speak up to tell my story. The instructor had read my book, knew my story of having died, and was given another chance to live. He knew what I should have been talking about. I was so nervous; I was failing this class big time!

During the last class when it was my turn for the final mock interview, I sat down and felt as if I was on worldwide television. As usual, I was shaking terribly and reluctant to speak.

Joel reached over, took my hand in his, looked me straight in the eyes and said, "Joyce, I want to ask you a question. Do you think God sent you back with a message?"

Boldly and confidently, I replied: "Yes HE did!"

Joel then said firmly, "Do you think your humbleness is getting in the way of God's message?"

I answered adamantly, "Yes it is!" At that moment I felt empowered, determined, and enthusiastic to share God's message with all who would listen about the importance of making it through problems rather than giving up because of them, and how to make certain we enjoy the Other Side when we get there.

Joel then proceeded to interview me as if I were on different types of talk shows that made up for all my previously failed interviews during these classes. At the end, we each were given a form to write an ad about our books that would be seen by radio talk show producers so they could decide if they wanted to invite us to be on their talk show.

As I was about to leave, Joel gave me the following quote to put on the back of my book: "Dr. Joyce Brown is a hugely inspiring human being… you are bound to be moved by her book and by her."

Also, he said I could be on any talk show in America, and added with a laugh, other than "Howard Stern."

On my drive home from that final class I felt this continued and enlivened passion and purpose to share God's message of the importance of using our limited Earth time wisely to make certain we enjoy the Other Side when we get there. I knew this message would save and change countless lives.

CHAPTER 56

The Howard Stern Show

The following week I received my first call from the ad I had previously filled out at the class for authors.

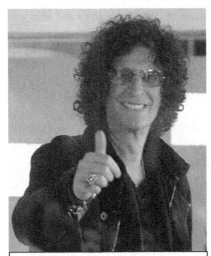

American radio and television personality Howard Stern. Photo: Bill Norton.

When I realized who it was, my eyes popped, my jaw dropped, and my heart began pounding. The man on the phone was a producer, and he invited me to be a guest on Howard Stern's Live Drive-by Show! At the time, Howard Stern's show aired in 60 markets and attracted 20 million listeners.

Even though I was shocked, amazed and apprehensive, knowing millions of listeners heard this show; I controlled my voice and sounded enthusiastic as I bravely accepted.

Immediately afterwards, I began asking other Christian authors if I should go through with this interview. They all told me "yes" and that it may be the only time that Howard Stern's audience might hear my unique message from God.

The producers soon contacted me to make arrangements for our interview to be broadcast live on Howard Stern's coast to coast radio show.

My interviewing skills that I had learned in the class were particularly useful in helping me change his "Howard Stern-type questions" to talk about heaven and the Other Side.

For example, he asked me if they have sex in heaven. I quickly pivoted, and replied, "What I learned on the Other Side was how important it is to use our limited Earth time wisely. And that there are things we can do here while we are still alive to make certain we enjoy Heaven when we get there."

Although it was a great opportunity, it was such a relief when it was over. I was glad that I had this rare and special invitation, and shared my experience and my message with him and his audience.

Over the years, I have to chuckle when people find out and say to me, "*YOU* were on *the Howard Stern Show?*"

CHAPTER 57

Stress and Grief Relief, Inc.

My passion for saving lives continued to increase. I decided I wanted to form a non-profit organization, and maintain a suicide hotline (877) 375-6923 (877-DR-JOYCE).

A life-Changing, Life-Saving Organization

In 1999, I founded Stress and Grief Relief, Inc., a 501(c)(3) non-profit organization dedicated to changing and saving lives, preventing suicide and its causes. This is a non-denominational, non-partisan, life-changing and life-saving public charity.

With God's help and direction, I met an extremely knowledgeable Enrolled Agent named Jim Quick, who previously helped organize and file multiple non-profits that became some of the top in the nation. Some still feed millions in the world.

Jim Quick is an amazing, caring, and God-loving man. He helped us fulfill all of the requirements of registering our non-profit with the Internal Revenue Service (IRS), making us eligible for tax-deductible donations, as well as keeping us current with all of the yearly forms and requirements.

Jim has become a dear friend to me. Many of my challenging days have been brightened by Jim's perfectly apt quotes from the Bible.

Even though I believe in God and share my story when I have the opportunity, and when it is appropriate, we work with people from all walks of life, and personal beliefs.

Over the years, I've worked with people of all different faiths. What they all believed in is the importance of using our Earth time wisely and making the best of each day.

Along with a variety of different religious beliefs, and beliefs about God, everyone is at their own individual level of growth. In some places it is not even legal or acceptable to speak about God. As counselors, coaches, and motivational speakers, we work with everyone according to their own specific needs and beliefs.

This book is also about my own life's journey, the promise I made to God about helping others, and my desire to make certain we enjoy the Other Side when we get there.

CHAPTER 58

False Promise, Real Fire

After we started the non-profit organization, a supposedly honest, religious person arranged for us to receive a donation of a mortgage note on twelve apartments for $250,000. The note was from a third party whose foundation needed to donate to a non-profit in 2001. This would have provided us with an income. After the donation to our non-profit was completed, this individual forged some documents, putting the note and mortgage from the third party in his *own* name so that *he* could collect the rents and live in one of the apartments for free. In essence, he defrauded us of the foundation's note which deprived our non-profit of the income from the apartments.

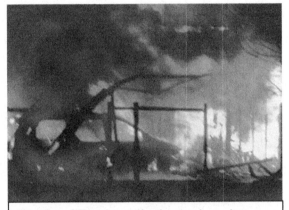

Photo of Dr. Joyce's three-alarm house fire which was printed in the local newspaper (you can see the outline of the car rental in front).

Over the next few years, we battled in court, which cost high attorney's fees, but we finally won. However, the court costs ate up more than the ultimate recovery. The court finally ruled in our favor in 2006. We technically won, yet somehow, they managed to create more and more horrendous court battles that continued and didn't settle until November of 2019; meanwhile, I still had all of the other stressful situations going on in my life.

Also in 2006, within 24 hours of trying to foreclose on the property with the twelve apartments that he had taken over, the house I'd previously built and lived in for many years in another state was burned down.

Was it just a coincidence?

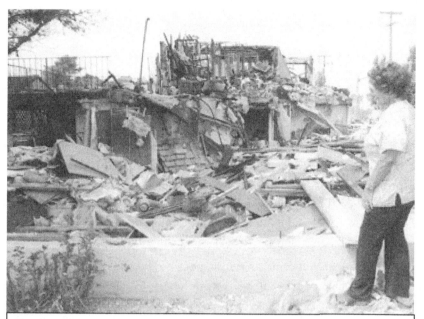

Dr. Joyce surveying the damage, searching for any valuables or documents. Sadly, the thieves were almost as bad as the fire.

The house fire was ruled as set by an unknown arsonist. When the court case was finally settled at the end of 2019, we found out that he had admitted to several people that he did arrange for my house to be set on fire; however, he died a few years before, and one of his associates was continuing the battle in his name.

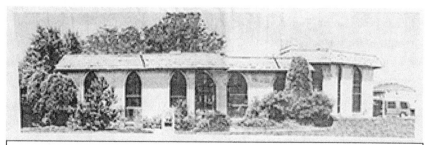

Dr. Joyce's home before the fire.

CHAPTER 59

Grief Relief and a Visit from the Other Side

In late June of 2003, I answered the phone and was surprised to hear that my half-sister, Shirley, was found dead. For years, she had been battling depression. Almost monthly, we had discussions by phone, during which I reminded her of reasons she should live. She always seemed to refer to the fact that our father had committed suicide, and that if it was good enough for him (she falsely believed), it was good enough for her.

Shirley's suicide came as a real shock to me, and I felt guilty that I hadn't been able to prevent it. Even though I'd been able to save many other people, I had not been able to save my own sister.

Daily for over a week, I cried and knelt at a particular rocking chair in my living room, asking for Shirley's and God's forgiveness, as I felt I had failed her. One day, as I was kneeling and praying with my head bowed, suddenly, over my left shoulder, I could see her clearly, with an otherworldly vision, even while my head was still bowed and my eyes were closed.

Sharply and firmly, she said, "Joyce, stop! I did this to myself! You always talk about using our time wisely, so stop crying, and grieving so much and move on with your life." Instantly, I felt a peace from God. I knew I was seeing her in a spiritual dimension, and that God and Shirley would work out whatever the consequences of her suicide would be, and that it was not my fault. However, I couldn't stop wondering what exactly Shirley meant when she said she did "this" to herself.

I remember seeing her in such clear and vivid detail. She was wearing a large, white T-shirt that came down past the middle of her thighs. From that moment on, I felt a new feeling of peace and realized that only God knows the intent of the heart, and only God can judge her actions.

About two months after her death, I received a phone call from a friend of hers who was the executor of her will, and was handling her estate. The woman informed me that my half-sister had left me a small gift.

Before we hung up, I asked her, "What was it with Shirley and a big white T-shirt?"

The lady gasped and said, "That was her favorite T-shirt. She loved that it was so big and comfortable, coming down to almost her knees. She was wearing it the day she died."

This was additional confirmation that God had allowed Shirley to come and tell me not to worry, to lift my grief, and to go on with my earthly life with heavenly peace, and without guilt.

CHAPTER 60

Expert Teachers, Exciting Times

In July of 2003, I received an unexpected call from my friend Irene Ross, who lived in California. We had both been very active in using and helping others with natural supplements, including those from a leading company with superb products, Nature's Sunshine. Irene invited me to come and stay with her and help with her holistic health clinic.

After a lot of study and work, I had received my license from the U.S. Department of Health and Human Services (HHS) as a qualified Naturopath, and I was looking forward to this new, unexpected opportunity to put this vital knowledge and wisdom into practical use.

In addition to helping Irene with her clinic in southern California, I was also excited to have the chance to take additional holistic health classes not available anywhere else.

Previously, I had had such a powerful, transformative learning experience with Dr. Jerry L. Tennant, MD, MD(H), PSc.D, who specializes in a unique healing methodology, that I was eager to discover additional healing

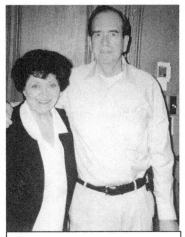

Dr. Joyce with Dr. Tennant at one of his specialized training programs.

modalities. The author of the wildly popular book *Healing is Voltage*, now in its 3rd edition, Dr. Tennant (see picture) continues to serve as an inspiration to me to this day, and I look forward to working with him whenever our schedules allow.

At the time, following my initial training with him, I turned my attention to additional healing methodologies that I could use to complement what I had learned from Dr. Tennant.

Since I was then in California, the next few weeks were jam-packed with special training from top doctors such as Dr. Bernard Jensen, and Dr. David Pesek. Given that I was now much closer to his practice south of the border, I also continued my custom-tailored training with Jose Antonio Calzada, M.D., H.M.D., who is a world renowned expert in stem cell therapy. Dr. Calzada has consulted with the National Olympic Committee regarding infectious diseases, including Zika, and he is an internationally recognized authority in alternative medicine.

Clearly, I was striving to ramp up and augment my knowledge and expertise as a Naturopath around this time, and I was thrilled to be learning from some of the top practitioners in the field. I soon began taking a variety of holistic classes, such as homeopathy, Ayurvedic medicine, enzyme therapy, and other natural health modalities with Melissa Welles-Murphy, another top holistic practitioner with clients and students from all over the world.

While staying in California, I was also doing some limited speaking engagements, and coaching. It seemed like my dreams were coming true, and I felt like I was on top of the world.

CHAPTER 61

A Dramatic, Lasting Change

Along with having learned and gained all this new knowledge and practical experience, 2003 turned out to be quite a year.

It was not only the year of my half-sister's suicide, but there was also a series of unexpected deaths of several close family members and dear friends.

Then, another disaster struck. I had been so busy throughout the holiday season that I had not been able to buy any gifts. So, on Christmas Eve, I decided to drive to the shopping mall. While stopped for the traffic in front of me, I leaned forward to try and see what was holding up traffic.

Suddenly, another car slammed into my van from behind. My head instantly snapped backward, and then forward, as my lower back jerked forward as well.

It turned out to be a three car crash. A crowd gathered around, and someone called an ambulance for me. I was more severely injured than the others. When the paramedics arrived they carefully strapped my head and back to a backboard. They believed my neck and back was broken.

When we arrived at the hospital they took X-rays and CAT scans. Doctors determined I needed to see a specialist not available in that area. With a lot of pain and difficulty, someone provided a ride back to where I was staying with Irene.

I wound up staying with my friend for another year. However, the auto accident crashed my dreams and plans with devastating and lasting physical limitations, and pain. To this day, I am still required to wear a back brace from this accident.

Even with all that I was enduring, I prayed constantly, asking God to help me adapt, and keep my eternal perspective. With determination and prayers, I was able to keep on doing what was essential: helping Irene, dealing with the lawsuits, and doing some coaching.

Before the accident, I had always been extraordinarily active, doing fun things like line-dancing, the jitterbug, and especially the twist, which I really enjoyed. I could really "cut a rug," let me tell you. Nevertheless, I continued striving to live life to the absolute fullest.

CHAPTER 62

Sharing the Stage With an Actress

In May of 2005, I went to a highly recommended health center in California, known for helping cases where others have given up. I had heard great things, and hoped they could help with my pain and inflammation. While I was there, I met a beautiful young woman who had severe stress and depression. During our conversations, I shared my book, told her about my near-death experience, and how important it is for each of us to find and pursue our own purpose for living.

She told me in detail of her definite plan to commit suicide. She felt anger, and held deep grudges against her parents, believing they had not taken proper care of her as a child. She felt her life was hopeless and that her death by suicide would teach them a lesson.

Over the next couple of days, I felt guided to help her understand the heart aches and challenges that her parents and grandparents had in coming from another country, changing cultures, and dealing with extreme financial hardships. I taught her how to meditate and how to feel calm, serene, and confident. She was also able to increase and improve her memory, which was critical to her work.

She quickly grasped these ideas and feelings and started to change her perspective, and her true, authentic personality burst forth like a blooming flower. With her depression gone, she was now both beautiful inside as well as outside. She was beaming as she told me she was looking forward to finding the right companion, getting married, and having children of her own. She said this would fit perfectly with her career as a movie actress.

She was thrilled with finding her new way of thinking, and her purpose for living. I hadn't recognized her because I rarely go to the movies, but during our conversations I learned others were aware that she was a well-known actress. She invited me to make arrangements to move to Beverly Hills to be her life coach. She reassured me there were others just like her who would like me to be their life coach also. This sounded exciting, and like a perfect fit.

CHAPTER 63

A Life Changing Phone Call

My thoughts of making a new life in Beverly Hills, and of being a mentor and coach for the young actress I'd met at the health resort were suddenly interrupted. I was notified by a staff member that I had an important phone call waiting for me at the front desk of the facility. Once again, my life and plans for the future were, without warning, dramatically changed.

It was from a cousin who explained she had responded to Mother's Life-Alert at 3 a.m., went to her apartment, and found her curled up under the kitchen sink. She was confused and obviously needed hospitalization.

For years, I tried to make sure I called my mom each morning and night to see how she was doing. Then she moved into a senior citizens' facility. Even when I was traveling, I still tried to call her twice a day. I made arrangements for her to wear a Life-Alert device around her neck. I also arranged for family and friends to regularly visit and check on her several days each week.

After I received that surprising phone call about my mother's deteriorating health condition, I knew that my phone calls and others checking on her were no longer adequate. I needed to be there.

My mother could no longer take care of herself. During her three days in the hospital of specialized care for diabetes and dementia, I had arranged for her to go into what I thought was a first-rate care facility where they could eat and socialize together. She was still somewhat independent and believed she was going to be getting married again, even though she was 90 years old. She had heard of rest home romances that had ended in marriage. She thought she might meet someone in this new facility. She was very petite, weighed about 79 pounds, had shrunk to about 4'6," and used a walker. She enjoyed visiting and was outgoing.

With her move to the care facility, I knew that I had to go home to personally make sure how she was doing and wanted to be there with her as much as I could. Though we had not gotten along well and had our challenges, she had given me life and brought me into the world, I knew it was my obligation and privilege to help her with her end of life care.

I had her medical power of attorney. She was on no medications, even for the diabetes. She just required small amounts of food often during the day. I gave explicit written, and witnessed, instructions that she was to receive no medication without my permission.

During this time, I was answering our non-profit suicide hot line, as well as keeping up with doctor's appointments regarding my back injuries. Being an N.M.D., I had patients call for advice including one who was in the emergency room who had just had an angiogram and was told he only had two weeks to live. As it turned out, after I worked with him and my doctors team helped him with alternatives to surgery, amazingly, he went on to live a much longer, productive life.

There was a lot going on in my life at the same time as I was taking care of my mother.

Her first couple of weeks seemed to go well. She was outgoing, happy and friendly. She sat in her chair in the doorway of her room and greeted people as they went by. This was in the first part of June. By the end of June, there were dramatic changes. I could tell she had lost weight and she was barely responsive when spoken to.

One morning when I went for my usual daily visit, I found my mother sitting in a little wheelchair in her room, gazing straight ahead. She didn't respond when I talked to her. She had a big, odd-looking bandage on the shin of her little leg. Feeling shocked and surprised, I asked the staff what had happened, but no one had an answer. They just shrugged off my questions and went back to work. I stayed with her until around 9:30 p.m. when I thought she would be safe for the night.

Over the next few days there were additional unexplained injuries and happenings. Even though I arrived by 9:30 a.m. each day, I couldn't imagine what was happening to her when I wasn't there. This was like a living nightmare. I couldn't find any of the staff members who would acknowledge that there was anything wrong.

I realized I needed to get her out of there and into another rest home. Frantically I searched for any information in finding a better place.

A couple of days later, with everything that was going on in my own life, the soonest I could get there was about 9 a.m. When I went into her room this time, I found her lying in bed, clinging to the bed rails, severely shaking with uncontrolled tremors, and she could not communicate with me. I could tell that she could hear me, but just could not respond.

There were state laws that had to be followed in order to transfer her to a different facility. This took about two weeks. It required a lot of hard work to find a better place that met all the state requirements before she could be transferred. I was with her from early morning to late at night.

I didn't know what they were doing, but I knew they were doing something to her. From within my heart and soul, I felt a desire and was compelled to sit in a chair by her bed and sing lullabies for hours. She could not communicate and was now like a little child. But I know she could hear me because unexpectedly, just as I finished one lullaby, she spoke up and said, "I know another one, '*A Little Birdie in a Tree.*'" Those were the last words she ever spoke.

Finally, we had met all the requirements and papers had been filled out; it was time for her to go to the new facility, Hazen Care Center. This new one was a wonderful, loving, caring rest home. The administrator/RN, Romaine Tuft, and her son, Greggory Tuft, arranged to come and get my mother. When they came in the room, Greggory, a husky young man, scooped Mother up, including her bedding. Mom wrapped her arms around his neck as he lifted her up. She was smiling as he carried her. She looked emaciated and I was grateful to get her out of there while she was still alive. We could tell Mother knew she was leaving this place and was very happy about it.

As we were leaving the old facility, the head nurse very begrudgingly gave us my mother's medical records.

What a change the new facility was. Everyone there was happy, well cared for, and seemed to feel contented. However, Mother's condition had deteriorated, and on the third day of our escape, I was so grateful to be sitting by her side when her eyes closed, a tear rolled down her cheek, and she passed to the Other Side.

I felt comforted knowing that when she died, people were around her who sincerely cared. I was so grateful that she did not die alone.

The administrator and head RN of the facility, Romaine Tuft, was so knowledgeable, and caring. She has become a lifelong friend.

During my mother's lifetime, she had helped many family members through their dire circumstances, people who had also lived during the Great Depression and were now already in Heaven. I knew she went home to a place where she had earned her peace of mind and was lovingly greeted by others who were already there. I'm sure they had a grand celebration for having made it through this mortal school of life.

Later, I learned a lot about good nursing homes and bad nursing homes. According to my mother's medical records, she had lost significant weight, down to 64 pounds. Also, contrary to my instructions, I discovered in her medical files from the old nursing home, that they had ordered five shots of Prolixen, a medication for out-of-control schizophrenics. I found out it should not be given to anyone over the age of 65, or under 90 pounds. My mother was 90 years old, and only weighed 64 pounds with her clothes on. My tiny mother was no danger to anyone.

Even though five injections had been ordered, she passed away after the second one. I believe this caused her death. I also found out the potential side-effects of this medication, and similar ones, can be severe shaking, trembling, inability to communicate, and depression. (This is known as Tardive Dyskinesia.)

After finding out about these types of rest homes and their use of medications to control patients, I have helped many others to make wiser choices for the care of their family members.

After her death, I was grieving severely and reminiscing over all the sad parts of my life. I was pleading with God to please help me get over this deep grief and pain and move forward with my life.

CHAPTER 64

Moving On

Meanwhile, the phone calls to the suicide hotline continued to come in with people desperately needing help. In time, my prayers were answered, and I was able to move on from the grief and pain of my mother's death.

In the fall of 2005, after having so many disappointments and sadness in my life, one day I received a letter which stated that I was being honored by the Utah Women's Alliance for Building Community. I learned later that I was being honored with the *first* Phyllis LeFevre Lifetime Community Builder Award in recognition of my work with community service programs, police departments, troubled youth, domestic violence, and suicide prevention. They said that my efforts made real and important differences in many communities and people's lives. The award would be presented at a banquet in October. It also invited me to a special luncheon before the event to meet with officers to get to know each other better.

I was surprised and delighted that I had won this prestigious award. I didn't know that anyone was even aware of all the work I was doing.

Later, while I was preparing to attend the banquet, my phone rang from our suicide hot-line. When I answered, I heard a frantic woman's voice say, "I know your organization, Stress and Grief Relief, is known for helping stop suicide. I desperately need your help right now. My brother called me and said that he has his finger on the trigger of his .45 revolver, pointed at his head, and when he pulls it, he will go to instant peace and wanted to tell me goodbye. He said he can't stand the pain after the loss of his wife."

The caller continued telling me she had called the police, who were at his door, but they didn't want to break in because they were concerned he might shoot them or himself. I told her, "Quick, give me his phone number."

This was back when they still had answering machines. I hoped that he might hear me as I was leaving a message. I dialed his number and after three long rings a voice came on that said, "This is John, goodbye to you and goodbye to the world, bury me in peace."

Believing he could hear me over the answering machine, I said, "Don't you want to know where you're going before you pull the trigger on that gun?"

"What if it's worse for you after you die than it is right now? How do I know? I used to be very suicidal. And then I actually died and went to the Other Side."

I kept talking into the recorder, hoping he was listening.

"I found out personally that it's not always nice there regardless of what we have done here on Earth. If suicide is a good idea," I said, "it will still be a good idea next week after you hear my story. Please let me just tell you about it."

Miraculously, what I said piqued his interest. He picked up the phone and gruffly said, "I will hear your story first. But if it's not what you say it is, I'm finishing the job."

He hung up the phone, let the police in, and they took him to a mental hospital.

That same night, I went on to the award ceremony with about 200 guests. I received a fantastic and heart–warming welcome. During my acceptance speech, I had another opportunity to tell my story of having been to the Other Side, discovering my life's purpose, and helping others to uncover their own purpose for living.

I was surprised and excited and felt like I was in another world. It was startling and almost overwhelming, but with their warm encouragement and congratulations, I was able to make a number of new friends.

Early the next morning, I made sure John received my book, *Amazing Heavenly Answers* at the facility where he'd been taken. In a short time, I found out that he had read my story, requested more books, and started a small suicide prevention group. Soon after he was released, he went back to school, continued his education, and earned his degree in psychology. And he kept on working in suicide prevention. Now John is saving lives.

CHAPTER 65

Life is Filled with Surprises

After being a widow for 7 ½ years, a friend arranged a blind date for me with a special man, Ron Runnells, who was retired. This friend believed we had mutual interests.

We had a storybook courtship filled with romance. After dating for a short time, one evening during a candlelight dinner, Ron proposed. It was very romantic and sweet. We felt like we were guided by God to be together at this time in our lives.

He knew about my near-death experience, and he understood and agreed that I needed to continue with my earthly mission. He knew that writing my book, *Heavenly Answers*, had been challenging, time consuming, and expensive to publish and distribute to those who needed it, and he understood that I would still keep my author's name, Joyce Hunt Brown.

He also knew I had founded a non-profit organization, Stress and Grief Relief, Inc, and that, along with counseling, a critical part of our strategic vision was (and remains) to get my books and audios out to as many people as we can, helping to prevent suicide and giving hope to the hopeless.

I explained to Ron that we needed to continue to raise funds and receive donations in order to distribute the books and sleep learning recordings in bulk to various groups—including prisons, centers for troubled youth, and individuals, as needed, as well as those who call the suicide hot-line, but also those who have started their own small groups around the book, helping others to overcome depression and find courage, faith, and their own true purpose for living.

After sharing the details around all of the work and expenses involved, I was so excited that Ron was actually looking forward to being a part of our cause, sharing God's message, and our unique coping techniques for stress, depression, grief, anger management, and suicide prevention throughout the world.

We married in January 2006.

My friends got together and gave us an outstanding reception; it was a luau, and included Polynesian entertainers, fire dancers, and fantastic food. Ron has a very special family, that mixed well with my family for this extraordinary occasion. We had two special official witnesses for our marriage ceremony, David W. Allan, the atomic clock scientist for the nation for 32 years, and D.J. Bawden, a well-known famous sculptor for Christian churches all over the world.

Prior to our marriage I knew, Ron, my husband to be, had extensive health problems. The doctors had given him two months to live due to severe heart and kidney problems. They wanted to insert a pacemaker.

However, with years of working with other top health specialists, successfully saving lives, and my own personal experience as a holistic health practitioner, I believed his life could be extended with help from God, holistic care and miracles.

A short time after Ron and I were married, my house was burned to the ground by an arsonist (as mentioned earlier). Ron and I happened to be on a trip in Nevada. This was the house I had built and lived in since 1973. The whole house was engulfed in flames that went over 65 feet in the air. It was what firefighters refer to as a *three-alarm fire*, a serious blaze requiring multiple trucks.

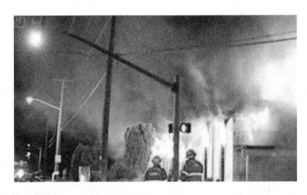

Shock, grief, sorrow and tears—a flood of emotions overwhelmed my entire body. I had just lost my entire home and most of what was inside, including heirlooms, and family keepsakes going back four generations.

In addition, all of my business equipment and records, along with my recording studio, were destroyed. If I had been in my house at the time of the fire, I probably would have died trying to save many of the important records and priceless mementos.

The insurance was inadequate to cover such priceless losses. This catastrophe, in addition to financial and health problems caused a level of grief that was challenging to overcome. In prayer, I felt heavenly whisperings that I would gain spiritually from this experience. However, my knowledge that problems are opportunities for mental and spiritual growth was severely tested.

Small Treasures Recovered and Lesson Learned

Day after day for several months, Ron and I dug through burned rubble hoping to salvage pictures, documents, and a few treasured mementos. Many times I quietly dried tears as I knelt in prayer and thanked God that my life had been spared. However, I could not let the debris be scooped up and hauled away until I looked through it all. Some of the pictures, notes, and correspondence that I found were priceless and worth the effort.

My famous gold-crowned tooth was found in the rubble, still intact, in the little brown prescription bottle where I had placed it years before. This became another great learning experience. My life since has been filled with miracles, insights, and loving relationships which became the heavenly stepping stones to the peace of mind and joy that I now have, which is more than I ever thought possible.

Along with this tragedy, shortly after the house fire, Ron's kidney problems worsened. The neurologist we went to insisted he needed a kidney removed. We made arrangements as soon as possible for his surgery.

After his operation, I discovered the doctor also removed a healthy adrenal gland in addition to the kidney. When I asked the surgeon why he removed a healthy adrenal gland, I was shocked when he said, "It was faster." He quickly turned, walked away, and began to talk to another patient.

When I had a health issue in the early 1960s, I was given some good advice. I had a good friend who was a general surgeon, and I asked him what I should do. He said, "There are answers, but don't ask a surgeon for a cure for a health issue. Their training and, therefore, their answer will be to have surgery." That certainly applied to Ron's kidney issue, and the removal of his healthy adrenal gland.

After Ron's recovery, we started working on rebuilding our lives. I may have lost my house and most everything in it, but at least we were both alive and able to start moving forward again.

Ron continued to receive specialized holistic health care which really helped his one remaining kidney and prevented him from needing a pacemaker. All of these holistic treatments ended up extending his life from the expected *two months*, given by top specialists, to the extra *ten years* of living with one kidney. It was yet another instance of how much one can still do even after all the doctors have said, "I'm sorry. Nothing more can be done."

After we were married, the next ten years of my life was an exceedingly difficult roller coaster. We had some precious good times, and my husband even enjoyed coming with me to some of my holistic health classes, before he had renal failure. Being a caregiver was extremely challenging, but we found ways to keep on keeping on.

In February of 2016, early one morning Ron awoke at about 5 a.m., took my hand in his and said, "I love you, Sweetie," then quietly passed to the Other Side. I became a widow again.

A few days before he passed, we had a talk about the realities of the Other Side, and not being able to communicate with someone, since they can actually hear us, but we can't usually hear them. With a heartfelt plea, I asked him, "If there is any way you can, please let me hear from you when you are on the Other Side."

A while after his passing, I felt prompted to put down some thoughts in the note app on my phone. I wrote, "Many times I'm confined to my reclining power chair. This past year my sweetheart died. Even though I am 83 years old, I am not giving up." Suddenly, a picture of his headstone from the graveyard, appeared between two sentences.

I went on and finished my notes. About a month later, while I was texting someone, who needed guidance and inspiration, another picture of Ron's gravestone appeared in the middle of the text.

Over the next three months, two more different pictures of his headstone appeared on my phone, for a total of four. I felt a feeling of peace from God for this blessing. I knew that Ron had succeeded in communicating with me and, in the process, touching my heart from the Other Side. This was comforting and helped me face the ordeals ahead.

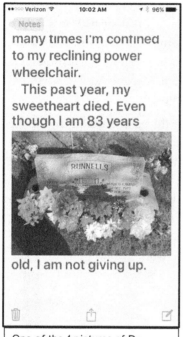

many times I'm confined to my reclining power wheelchair.

This past year, my sweetheart died. Even though I am 83 years

old, I am not giving up.

One of the 4 pictures of Dr. Joyce's deceased husband's headstone, which miraculously popped up on her phone.

For those who are grieving, I encourage you to be still and silent and try to listen to what your loved one may be trying to tell you.

Over the last two years of Ron's life he required almost constant care. After his passing I grieved extensively and really missed him. I was alone. The house seemed empty. I didn't want to go anywhere or do anything.

Though I was still grieving, I was able to arrange financing to cover the expenses of running the non-profit, including trade show displays, special health care events, key memberships, IANDS events and NSA meetings and workshops.

Life demands that we confront difficult situations. When people call me for grief relief after losing everything in a fire, or any other type of disaster, I am better able to feel empathy and counsel them as they make it through to build a new life.

Sometimes we are to change the situation the best we can. Other times, we must change ourselves.

We all grieve in our own way, even though there are many groups that are adamant that there are specific steps that someone must go through before they feel like going on with life. In my own case, having been a widow twice, and based on my own experience and grief counseling with many others, I know that this is not always true.

To be clear, it is *not* disrespectful to the person we've lost to make the most of our own limited Earth time. Based on my visit to the Other Side, I know that our loved ones would want us to move forward with our lives here on Earth.

What I learned from my near-death experience helped me to move ahead with my life. Whatever Earth time I had left was too short to stay stuck.

In the fall of 2016 and winter of 2017, I participated as a booth exhibitor with our non-profit organization, Stress and Grief Relief, Inc., at several health conferences and conventions. In addition, we had multiple meetings with those interested in near-death experiences and IANDS (International Association of Near-Death Studies).

All of these events required hiring many drivers and others to help me assemble and disassemble the displays. The exhibits proved to be highly effective. Along with other messages, the displays stated that we provide hope to those who feel life is not worth living, and for those who were seeking stress relief now. I was so excited to know that thousands of people were seeing our displays of hope, the importance of using Earth time wisely, and our pioneering ideas about how to learn while you sleep. I was certain the displays and the books that were given out were doing some good.

The meetings and conferences were fun, exciting, interesting, and, as I shared my story, they helped me to become a better messenger, with dramatic, uplifting results.

In part, because I am so eager and determined to spread God's message about how to make certain you enjoy the Other Side when you get there, I carry extra copies of my book wherever I go. It seems I

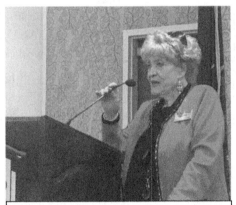

Dr. Joyce speaking at a Chamber of Commerce meeting.

always run into someone who has a need. Over the years, I've given away countless copies, in addition to those that are donated through our non-profit, Stress and Grief Relief, Inc.

As a result of always having extra copies of my books with me, and giving copies away to those in need, I have heard back from countless people, and learned of a number of interesting and miraculous stories of lives transformed.

CHAPTER 66

Finding Hope

My purpose and joy for living is to give hope to others, and an eternal perspective for living. This includes sharing my miraculous recovery from ALS, depression, and wanting to commit suicide, but also overcoming a number of other health crises and heartbreaking setbacks.

Life is filled with challenges and miracles. God is real. We grow and learn from tragedies and problems.

Many people are told their life is ending and nothing more can be done, as I was. Being given a death sentence is not necessarily the full story or the complete truth.

With the help of God, persistence and seeking natural health solutions, many lives are saved.

Because of natural medicine and devoted care giving, my recently deceased husband, Ron Runnells, lived 10 years longer than the doctors' prognosis and my previous husband, Earl Brown, lived 14 years longer than the doctors expected.

CHAPTER 67

Living a Life with Challenges, While Still Sharing Hope

Now at almost 90 years old, I am able to continue enjoying a busy lifestyle as I share what I learned while I was in Heaven during my near-death experience, and unique techniques for overcoming depression, anger, stress, and changing and saving lives.

Additionally, I feel driven to do all I can, while I can, which includes fulfilling speaking requests and interviews, conducting personal and group consultations, and continuing to write more books. Whenever and wherever possible, and appropriate, I share God's message of using our Earth time wisely.

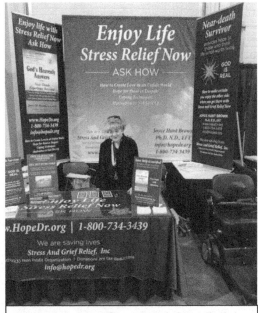

Dr. Joyce at her Stress and Grief Relief booth before one of the numerous trade shows.

Unfortunately, I still experience severe back pain from the auto accidents and failed back surgeries. In the summer of 2017, my doctor ordered multiple MRIs of my entire neck and back. Five compression fractures in my vertebrae were discovered. Additional areas of pressure on the spinal cord were also found, as well as three more herniated disks. These were new complications in the situation with my spine. The doctors were stunned and said that I could end up paralyzed or die at any time. By continuing to "keep on keeping on," I'm surprising them all.

Due to this condition, I can only walk short distances, and sit up for a limited time each day. This may slow me down, but it does not stop me. There are times when I need my reclining power chair in order to lie back. Then, whenever I need to go from place to place, I return it to its full upright position, or I jump on my Harley mobile. Regardless of how I move around, the fact is that most others still have trouble keeping up with me.

To be clear, despite the other challenges I have to navigate, I have not had any more symptoms of ALS since I was healed in 1988.

I do not dwell on what I cannot do. Instead, I feel forever grateful for the opportunities I have, and for new chances to learn and be of service.

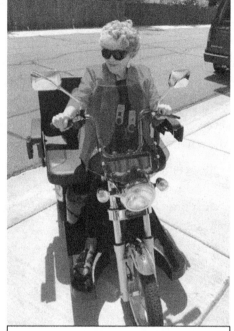

Dr. Joyce returning from an afternoon ride on her Harley mobile.

After many years of continued challenges and calamities in my life, in February of 2017, I finally found the time to rejoin the Las Vegas chapter of the National Speakers Association.

NSA Las Vegas has outstanding meetings, with training and coaching from remarkable speakers, including four International Toastmasters Champions—Mark Brown (1995), Craig Valentine (1999), Ed Tate (2000), and Darren LaCroix (2001)—as well as outstanding guest speakers from other chapters across the nation, such as Patricia Fripp, Michael Hauge, Ford Saekes, and Dan Clark. They all share their unique, motivational, life changing techniques.

I found it enlightening to hear about their particular methods of speaking to their audiences. This is helpful when I tell my story and the lessons I've learned. Since I've been applying what they taught, while being a part of the NSA group, not only am I reaching larger audiences, but more of my listeners are letting me know that they feel inspired and closer to God, and are coming up with good reasons to make it through their problems.

Each speaker has their own style for motivation with the end goal being to help each individual in their audience to find their purpose and improve their own lives.

At NSA they share their special methods with us, their fellow speakers. At every meeting there is always a new tip and information that I can apply to the way I share my story.

I've enjoyed mingling and getting to know a number of these people better. I love listening and learning from their stories and outstanding presentations. Several of these extraordinary people have become like family to me.

CHAPTER 68

Never Give Up

Even though only God can ultimately judge someone's actions, my visit to the Other Side showed me just how important it is to not give up on life, but also for each of us to find our own true purpose for living. This can bring feelings of zest and joy. It also helps in overcoming problems and attaining peace of mind for ourselves and others. As we live our purpose optimistically, with prayer, courage, and faith, rather than giving up, we are more apt to receive miracles, and enjoy the Other Side when we get there. Using the power of "positive belief," we can change our self-talk which can change our lives.

I know there are some people who say it does not matter how we live our lives, or how we use our Earth time. However, what if it does make a difference? Remember what the Bible says: "Do unto others as you would have them do unto you." Also, "Love thy neighbor as thyself." Putting these simple truths into practice will bless many lives and can create miracles for ourselves and others.

My personal experience dispels the myth that just by dying you can automatically receive peace of mind, regardless of how you've lived your life.

Our time here on Earth is too valuable to waste. I am grateful for what I can still do and accomplish each day. Prayer, wisdom, and inspiration help guide us through our lives. What a difference the world would be if we could all be more Christ-like.

Over the years, I have had a wide variety of opportunities to share God's message and His heavenly answers for us all. When people tell me their success stories, it touches my heart, and they become my mental cheerleaders. I feel energized with joy and peace in my soul as I continue trying to fulfill my purpose for living as I promised God I would do.

CHAPTER 69

My Journey Through Blindness

In November of 2011, even though I had been getting injections in my eyes since 2009, my vision was totally lost. It was so far gone, in fact, that I needed a flashlight to see a glass of water at my side. I was told by eye specialists that I had both dry and extreme wet macular degeneration and that my vision would never get better since it had suddenly gotten so much worse, even after all the injections.

Normal vision is 20/20, but legally blind is 20/200. When asked to read the eye chart, I couldn't even see the chart. The assistant pulled up a chair in front of me. She held up her fingers and said to tell her when I could see them. I couldn't see anything until her fingers were below her shoulders. Then I could barely make out two fingers in my peripheral vision. I asked her if anyone had ever gotten their vision back when it had progressed to this point.

She answered, "I'm sorry, no."

I said with faith, "Then, I will be the first."

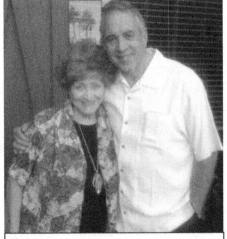

Dr. Joyce with Bill Sardi, "The Vitamin Supplement Answer Man."

At the time, I'd had injections in each eye to supposedly slow down the bleeding in both retinas. Unfortunately, after over 70 injections it still had not worked.

I had heard resveratrol could help with vision. I had also previously taken eight different supplements with various brands of resveratrol, but was disappointed that none of them made any difference.

In 2012, I was introduced to Bill Sardi, an expert in all aspects of improving vision, health, nutrition and living a longer healthier life. Known as the "Vitamin Supplement Answer Man," Bill had the perfect solution for my problem, an effective natural supplement, Longevinex, which includes a special formula and type of resveratrol. He sent it to me overnight.

Surprisingly, after taking it for just a few days, my vision was miraculously restored to the point I could thread a needle. I was also able to renew my driver's license.

Shortly thereafter, the story of my vision being restored was covered in-depth by the Emmy and Peabody award-winning journalist George Knapp on CBS News.

In June 2013, the National Academy of Television Arts and Sciences awarded George Knapp and KLAS with an Emmy for their story about my restored vision using Longevinex, entitled *Miracle Eye Cure*.

However, even though my vision restoration was miraculous, the number of injections was misstated as only being 17, when it actually had been over 70, which was even more miraculous. But it was too late to fix it after the story was published and distributed.

I was excited when Bill Sardi invited me to a luncheon in Las Vegas to meet Dr. Stuart Richer O.D., Ph.D., President of the Ocular Nutrition Society. I learned that Dr. Richer had been working with multiple patients who had macular degeneration who got their vision back after taking Longevinex®.

In fact, referring to Longevinex, Dr. Richer writes, "Macular degeneration affects millions of senior adults. There is no proven remedy for this insidious sight-robbing disease. The fact that a nutraceutical (Longevinex®) has been demonstrated for the first time to reverse a predictive measure for macular degeneration is a monumental development in preventive medicine."

Unfortunately, over a few years, I developed some new and very serious vision problems because of scarring from the previous extensive bleeding in my retinas, prior to taking the resveratrol supplement.

As bad as my vision problem is today, it is still not nearly as bad as when my vision was totally *gone* because of severe wet macular degeneration. If only I had known about and taken Longevinex earlier, I know I would not have had any macular degeneration in the first place.

It's my belief anyone over the age of 60 should take Longevinex® as a needed health supplement to prevent age related macular degeneration. I strongly suggest you call the Longevinex® office, ask for information about the product and request their newsletter which has tremendously helpful health information not found anywhere else. Bill Sardi personally writes the newsletter. It's exceptionally informative and helps us understand how to improve our health at the cellular and even molecular level.

There was another episode in my life that convinced me of the importance of continuing to take Longevinex. During my doctor's visits in 2017, when I was told I could become paralyzed or die at any time because of the severe pressure on my spine, I felt shocked. When I came home, I was still in shock. There were other things in my life that took priority with my limited time, and I overlooked taking any of my supplements. I began to concentrate on other things that seemed to be more important.

However, about a month before, since it had been nearly three years since I had my eyes checked, I had made a new appointment. This was after receiving the bad news from the previous doctor, who had given me the shocking news about my spinal condition.

When I went to the eye specialist, and while they were examining deep inside my eyes with their special equipment, the doctor said, "Oh, your left eye is hemorrhaging in the retina."

As he said that, I realized I'd forgotten to take my Longevinex® during the past few weeks. I spoke up quickly and asked for another appointment for him to check it again in two weeks. After I arrived home, I immediately got back on my daily resveratrol regimen.

Two weeks later, when I returned for my appointment and the doctor rechecked my eyes, he was surprised and said, "The hemorrhaging has stopped."

With a sound of utter disbelief, he repeated, "There is no more bleeding in your retina."

I could tell he was astonished. He seemed very perplexed, but he did not ask why. I tried to tell him about Longevinex, but he was too busy to listen.

This experience reinforced my determination to take the resveratrol supplement *every day*. I also take it because I've had heart problems for years. I've read scientific studies on animals which demonstrate that Longevinex can reduce the size of a heart attack (as measured by scar tissue), reduce the death of heart muscle cells, double the heart pumping pressure, and increase the blood flow in the aorta (*Health Freedom News, Winter 2017*).

Back in 2012, I had my husband Ron start taking Longevinex for his slow and irregular heartbeat (atrial fibrillation, often referred to as "A-Fib"), which, at the time, he had had for more than 25 years. The body is electrical, and when it gets out of balance it can cause health problems such as irregular heartbeat. As a result of Bill Sardi's recommendation, Ron took Longevinex, water-soluble B1, and Magnesium. He did not need a pacemaker as his physicians had previously proposed. Not only did the A-Fib completely disappear, but it also significantly improved his heart condition, and even improved his vision.

Dr. Nathaniel Lebowitz, a physician specializing in preventive cardiology, also stands behind resveratrol and this particular resveratrol supplement. In fact, he has stated, "A particular brand of resveratrol, Longevinex, is recommended to our patients because it is the only brand that has been shown to reduce damage to the heart better than plain resveratrol in experimental animal studies. I've been recommending a resveratrol pill for my patients for over a decade now. Among all the medicines I use," Lebowitz continues, "this dietary supplement is the one that has the most promising science behind it."

I am also aware of studies that have shown Longevinex has an anti-aging benefit, enabling people to live longer, healthier lives.

Even though I have some vision problems now, it is much better than the total vision loss I had in November 2011. With the continued use of resveratrol, it has stopped the bleeding for over eight years. I've not required any more injections since then, even though the doctors previously told me I would have to have them for the rest of my life.

The low vision I have now is caused by the *scarring* from the previous bleeding from years ago. Had I known years ago what I know now, I believe these vision problems could have been prevented.

I am aware of and have personally tried thousands of dollars of low vision products, most of which did not work for me, but may work for others, and still additional products which are just false promises or scams.

I know of numerous other people who have had miraculous results with their vision using this particular product. I faithfully use Longevinex, and regularly recommend it, but I do not sell it. Of course I cannot promise what it will do for others, but it's worked wonders for me and many others I know personally. I believe it is only available directly from the company. For more information, visit Longevinex.com.

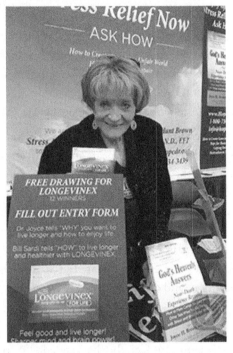

As I often share whenever I conduct health workshops, host a booth at a health fair, or do health counseling, as much as I can I share info about Longevinex®. In fact, as a bonus, I hold drawings for free boxes of Longevinex®. As I often say, Bill Sardi has the story about "how" to live longer, and I have the story about "why" to live longer.

This has been another part of my life's journey of finding hope and miracles which I often share with those who are having vision problems.

CHAPTER 70

Finding Peace of Mind

My soul still yearns to share with family, friends, and the whole world, regarding the importance of making it *through life's problems*, rather than quitting life because of them. Whenever and wherever possible, I have related my personal story and the potential eternal benefits or consequences of utilizing our Earth time wisely.

I feel heartfelt gratitude that numerous people have responded to my message. I have received miraculous accounts and priceless personal stories.

Many, including their family members, have expressed gratitude for receiving a new Other Side perspective for living. They are now helping to share God's message, to "keep on keeping on," despite the countless challenges they face here on Earth.

The good news is, with God's grace and in His timing, survivors of those who have lost a loved one *can* find peace and comfort to continue their own individual life's journey.

I feel immense joy when I hear back from others who have overcome their negative attitudes, feel better about the life they're now living, hope to have a more pleasing life review when they are on the Other Side, and feel better prepared to meet God when their time comes.

The following are just a handful of examples of the type of responses I have received. Perhaps you may know someone who is struggling with similar problems and may benefit by learning eternal truths, and from other's success stories.

More Letters from Readers

"I will forever be grateful to Dr. Joyce for saving my youngest daughter's life. When she found evidence that suggested her husband was cheating on her, she overdosed on meds and attempted to take her life. After hours in a coma, the medical personnel were able to bring her around.

She was devastated that her suicide attempt had failed and was absolutely determined to try again, someplace where she wouldn't be found in time.

"Feeling helpless, I brought her to my home and gave her Dr, Joyce's book, Heavenly Answers to read. While I didn't expect her to, she did, indeed read it, and her whole attitude changed. She was able to call Joyce, who was willing to have long conversations with her. She had a small son at the time who really needed his mommy, so what a blessing it was to her loved ones that she was willing to read that book and accept help!

"Now, several years later, she is a happy homemaker, stressed with medical problems like MS, but determined to hang in there and make the most of what she has been dealt. So, thank you with all my heart, Dr. Joyce Brown!"

"PS: I never did learn if her husband really was unfaithful, but he's very devoted to her since."

—Lily Palmer

"This book is a self-contained support system."

—Karen Anderson

"A friend gave me Dr. Joyce Brown's book. To pacify her, I agreed to read a few pages, although I had definitely decided to commit suicide that day—my suicide note was already written. But I couldn't put the book down. I then saw my world from a new perspective and wanted to share this life-changing, life-saving, near-death account with loved ones and friends. The next day I ordered 20 books to give out to friends and family."

—Helen Johnson

These are just a few samples of the many letters I have received letting me know of the countless lives that were changed after hearing and applying God's messages.

We all make mistakes in our lives. However, even if someone's yesterdays are scarlet, with God's help their tomorrows can be snow white.

It is my hope and prayer that by telling my life story, including eternal truths, it will cause a ripple effect throughout the world for many generations to come.

It is important that we use our Earth time wisely. There *is* life after life. We *can* make certain we enjoy the Other Side when we get there.

As author and composer Janice Kapp Perry said about the first edition of *Heavenly Answers*, "The day after I read this book…I viewed my life from a completely different, and much improved perspective. It's great to be reminded in such a compelling way about what matters most—now and in eternity."

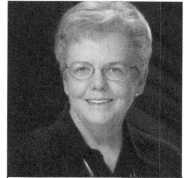

Prolific American composer, songwriter, and author Janice Kapp Perry.

CHAPTER 71

Believe in Miracles

Many times, people ask me, "Why have you had so many problems?" I always tell them, "We develop physical muscles by lifting weights. We develop mental and spiritual muscles by overcoming problems or making it through setbacks and challenges without giving up."

It may not have seemed like it at the time, but by making it through problems, they became opportunities for me to learn and grow. As I made it through challenges, each of them helped me develop empathy, and gain the ability to better help others going through similar situations. Ultimately, the difficulties became a blessing in disguise.

With sincere prayers, I want to be a true messenger, and keep sharing God's eternal truths. Life is too short to be easily offended, angry, have self-defeating thoughts, or hold grudges.

As I said before, it is important to become Christ-like, loving, kind, forgiving and merciful, *especially while driving.*

Since I am in my ninth decade and do not know how much more time God will grant me, I am having a bench made for my grave with my message to the world:

Our Lord God Is Real! Now is not forever.
Life is a journey, not a destination,
Love life and others.

Remember: We can create miracles for ourselves. If you have been diagnosed with ALS, or any other illness, and the doctor says, "nothing more can be done," keep searching for physical, mental, and spiritual solutions until you find what works for you.

One of my favorite sayings is: *Believe in Miracles, Expect Miracles, Be a Miracle for someone else.*

CHAPTER 72

Looking Back on My Life's Journey

In my struggles for health, to live, to walk, to see, to succeed, I have had to overcome what seemed like impossible obstacles by worldly standards. With the help of God, I have endeavored to painstakingly build the obstacles into heavenly stepping-stones of understanding more thoroughly what this life is all about. I am trying to fulfill my real purpose in life: caring and sharing.

As I look back now at almost 90 years old, I realize gratefully, with God's help, I made it through so many different trials and tribulations throughout my life, including ALS, Myasthenia gravis, terrible auto accidents, failed back surgeries, agoraphobia, depression, the death and loss of loved ones, a devastating house fire at the hand of a bitter arsonist, my own struggles with thoughts of suicide, as well as the loss of my father, sister, and others to suicide.

I can now see that as I searched and pleaded for solutions to my problems, I gained knowledge, wisdom, and information that can truly help me and many other people.

In fact, going through these many difficult challenges, losses, and setbacks led me to create our non-profit organization, Stress and Grief Relief, Inc. A vital part of this is work is helping those struggling with the loss of a loved one—particularly those who are grieving after the suicide of a family member or friend—so they can find hope, Heavenly peace of mind, and move forward with their own lives. I truly understand how they feel.

Death is not the end. There is life after life. Again, it is so important to understand that your loved ones, when they die, they become your spiritual cheerleaders and want you to make the most of whatever Earth time you have left. None of us know for sure if we have a tomorrow.

I also learned that our pets go to heaven, receive peace and joy, and we will see them again as well. Having just recently lost my constant 9-year-companion, Kitty, this is a subject close to my heart. In fact, I have begun writing a new book entitled, *The Secret Life of My Little Service Dog Named Kitty and Proof She Went to Heaven*.

I also reaped countless miracles. At almost 90 years old, I am truly a transformed person.

We are here to "learn the lessons of life." The wisdom I've acquired while going through trials, challenges and calamities have cost me dearly. My soul's sincere desire is to share with all who want to improve their own mental and spiritual well-being. We need to care for our lives, we need to care for our planet. There are ways and means to attain a better quality of living with courage, faith and hope.

My quest for answers has taken me to the far corners of the world. I have been privileged to visit the legendary "Holy Mountains" and even the mysterious "Lost Caves." I was blessed to be given the opportunity to work with top scientists, world-recognized engineers, and internationally acclaimed physicians. I have researched and explored both modern and ancient manuscripts and have discovered some of the greatest eternal truths of the ages.

Yes, my life has been blessed with miracles, but I had to *reap* them. Over the last 80-plus years, my life has been a miraculous journey. I enjoy teaching others how to reap miracles too!

Each of us can be more, have more, and do more for ourselves, and others, and for this world. We can have a happier life, and a cleaner environment. We can grow rich mentally and spiritually. We can have more time for fun, profit, and for reaping miraculous results.

American clergyman Edward Everett Hale wrote in *The Power of One*, "I am only one, but still, I am one. I cannot do everything, but still, I can do something. And because I cannot do everything, I will not refuse to do the something that I can do." As I share my message with those who want to listen, I believe we can all do something to help make this world a better place. Whatever we can do, with the help of God, if we *will* do it, we can make this a better world for us all.

What I sincerely desire is success—not success the way the world defines it, but success the way Ralph Waldo Emerson defined it in his 1909 essay, *Success*:

"To laugh often and much;

To win the respect of intelligent people and the affection of children;

To learn the appreciation of honest critics and endure the betrayal of false friends;

To appreciate beauty,

To find the best in others;

To leave the world a bit better, whether by a healthy child, a garden patch or a redeemed social condition;

To know even one life has breathed easier because you have lived.

This is to have succeeded."

How to Have an Awesome Day

For Now

I will be cheerful, loving and kind.

For Now

I will try to adjust myself to what is; Not try to adjust everything
to my own desires.

For Now

I will speak softly, be calm, patient, and forgiving.

For Now

I will do a good turn or a kind deed.

For Now

I will be as agreeable as I can.

For Now

I will try to live through this day only.

For Now

I will give myself at least a half hour for meditating,
counting my blessings and giving thanks for what I have.

For Now

I will have faith, be confident and express gratitude.

For Now

I will look for the good in everyone and everything.

For Now

I will remember to breathe deeply and smile often.

*"Every adversity carries with it seeds of benefits—the challenge is to 'keep on keeping
on' until we find the benefits."*

~ Dr. Joyce

Book Summary by Kimberly Clark Sharp, M.S.W., Author of *After the Light*

For anyone who has ever toyed with the notion of "ending it all" in an attempt to go to the place of love and light, Joyce Brown offers an important reality check. There is a *reason* why we are here and why our life is not over, no matter how bleak our current situation may be. Immense rewards—spiritual rewards—await those of us who persevere in the face of trials and try our best to learn and to grow.

In my own book, I wrote: "The Light was brighter than hundreds of suns but did not hurt my eyes. I immediately understood it was entirely composed of love, all directed at me. I was with my Creator, God, in holy communication. The Light gave me knowledge that I seemed to be remembering rather than learning, and included answers to questions that any fool would ask in the presence of the Almighty. 'Why are we here?' *To learn.* 'What's the purpose of our life?' *To love.* And, among other questions, 'What about suicide?' The answer I understood was, *'If you didn't create it, you can't destroy it.'* I took that as advice to not deliberately end our Earthly lives prematurely. Why not? Well, if life is a metaphor for school, consider that if we drop out in say, March, we cannot at such time as we figure out we need more education, begin again in March. We have to repeat the entire school year and probably have to take remedial classes. We end up working harder than if we had stuck it out in the first place."

I wish I had been able to convince Joyce Brown of this earlier in her life, but then she would have missed the most remarkable experience of her life.

After a prolonged and serious illness with debilitating pain, Joyce Brown willed herself dead. She had a near-death experience, but it was not what she expected. Instead of bliss and blessedness, she had an "extremely anguishing experience" wherein she suddenly realized all that she had lost by giving up on life. The wispy spiritual body she now possessed could not speak to her loved ones or pick up pen and paper to write them. She was overwhelmed by a desperate longing for her pain-racked Earthly body as she realized that she could no longer communicate to her family how much she loved and missed them. She had her chance at Earthly life and now it was over.

But fortunately for us, it wasn't over. A "beautiful Being of Light" ushered her into His presence and began to teach her about life. She saw that life is like a race and that it is important to continue that race until its natural end. The barriers and obstacles that we encounter on this race are there to help us learn and grow.

She was shown the agonies of people who had ended their lives early and who then tried desperately and without success to warn others who were present at their funerals. She came to know that there is no such thing as "ending it all" and that the problems people face may even get worse when they terminate their lives before their time.

She learned how people who appear to "have it all" really don't and why we would not want to trade places with those who seem to float through life unscathed by problems. She was taught why we have the problems we do and how we can learn from every situation, no matter how difficult.

Then she saw that rich rewards and priceless joys await many of the most humble people on Earth who valiantly suffer through their trials and tribulation. Fortunately for whiners such as myself, complaining while suffering is okay.

She witnessed intense marital arguments from inside the mind of each participant and could see that what they were saying did not correspond with how they were really feeling. She saw the utter futility of bitter, heated disputes and learned how such conflicts could be resolved. She also saw a miserable place for souls who died while still holding onto their spiteful grudges.

Accordingly, Joyce came to understand that any deed we do with unrighteous motivation or intention actually hurts ourselves. On the other hand, forgiveness—whether requested or not, whether deserved or not—brings heavenly rewards beyond comprehension.

In summation, the things we say and do on Earth can drain or build our character and spiritual strength with results that show up when we arrive on the Other Side. The way Joyce figures it, we are literally building a heavenly retirement fund!

When confronted with the question, "In life, what did you do with what you had?" none of the carefully crafted excuses that had previously shielded Joyce from accepting responsibility for who she was and how she acted had any effect. In re-experiencing everything that happened in her life, she realized we "score" simply by how well we do with what we have.

She learned that miracles are actually common and happen more easily for those who believe in them. She was surprised that more of her prayers had been answered than she realized and that she had been blessed many times without knowing it. She also saw the difference in how beauty is created and valued on Earth and how beauty is created and valued on the Other Side. Her insights reinforce the timeless truths from Jesus' Sermon on the Mount.

Joyce Brown asks us to please hear her message: *Life is Worth Living!* I agree with my whole heart. There is a peace in knowing that a great leveling is coming, that every valley shall be exalted and every mountain and hill made low, that people who lead lives of challenge and heartache have greater growth opportunities than those who have lives of ease; that this is our chance to learn and grow spiritually, to experience and accomplish things that can only take place in an Earthly existence.

We get up from reading this book grateful to be alive and to have the chance afforded by each day to do good and to be good. There is power in the lessons of this book, power that the least of us can use in meeting the challenges that come to us every day.

This book is about life and afterlife. It helps us understand the big picture—why we are here and why life unfolds as it does—and it helps us gain strength for the daily challenges we all face as long as we exist in Earthly form. Life indeed is worth living and *Amazing Heavenly Answers* helps us understand our personal purpose and path.

About the Author

Dr. Joyce Hunt Brown has had an interesting and challenging life. After a lifetime of heartbreaking tragedies, the great turning point of her life arrived. A two-year period of being bedridden and deathly ill culminated in a profound near-death experience in 1983. Now equipped with a wealth of heavenly answers for earthly challenges, this was the transforming incident where she went from desperately wanting to die, to desperately wanting to help others live.

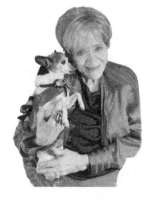

Unfortunately, the major life challenges were not over. After experiencing severe health problems for some time, including losing her voice, Dr. Joyce was diagnosed with ALS in 1988, at the age of 54. Following a miraculous recovery from ALS, including regaining an even more youthful voice, her doctors were left dumbfounded while Dr. Joyce doubled down on her desire to help people turn stress into success.

In fact, since then, across the nation and around the world, Dr. Joyce has been working energetically, answering calls, training groups and organizations, and, in the process, saving and transforming lives. She has brought innumerable people back from the brink of suicide, depression, and grief. She has helped people overcome anger, anxiety, and chronic stress. Through her ongoing work as a guest speaker and trainer, she has a long record of helping organizations strengthen morale, improve communication, resolve conflict, and increase productivity.

As a certified crisis chaplain, Dr. Joyce also continues to visit with groups of teens at youth detention centers, inmates at prisons, various different groups in churches, and at-risk kids in schools. To continue this work Dr. Joyce founded Stress and Grief Relief, Inc. a 501(c)(3) non-profit, public charity in 1999.

Making frequent guest appearances on television as "The Hope Doctor," Dr. Joyce is the host and producer of The Hope Doctor Show, where she shares from her remarkable story, and the eternal wisdom that radically transformed and gave new meaning and purpose to her life. This wisdom includes the unique methods and proven techniques she utilizes in helping people and organizations thrive and strive for miraculous success.

Known as a trusted advisor and "the Therapist's Therapist," Dr. Joyce is an author, speaker, coach, and Certified Crisis Chaplain. She is also a Board-Certified expert and Diplomate with the American Academy of Experts in Traumatic Stress®. While in practice as a Naturopathic Medical Doctor (N.M.D.), Dr. Joyce received six Lifetime Achievement Awards in the natural health field. She is the author of the books *Amazing Heavenly Answers*, *Near Death Survivor Conquers ALS, Depression, Grief, Suicide & More: A Book of Hope*, as well as the sleep learning audio recordings, *Whispers for Life and Prosperity* and the specialized meditation, *Whispers for Miraculous Results*. Some of her most popular programs include:

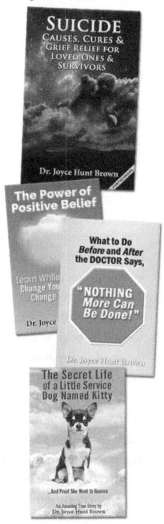

1. *The Power of Positive Belief: Change Your Self-Talk, Change Your Life*
2. *Super Goals: Desire, Visualize, and Realize Miraculous Results*
3. *The Ultimate Mindset: Unleash the Power of Your Miraculous Mind.*

Her websites are: www.HopeDr.org and www.StressAndGriefRelief.org

Pay It Forward

Keep the Message Going

Depression is a very serious problem in our nation (and worldwide). Hopelessness is rampant, and suicides continue to plague our world. ***But there is hope!***

Our organization is devoted to stopping suicides and overcoming depression. Every year, MANY people are given HOPE, LOVE, and PEACE, and decide to begin really living! My book, *Amazing Heavenly Answers*, has proven to be the catalyst that brings true hope and change to many lives.

I pray that this book will continue to be an influence for good to those who feel overwhelmed and stressed by life and to those who mistakenly long for the peace of death. I especially pray that it will restrain those who may be contemplating ending their own lives.

We provide the book free of charge for those who need it, and to support groups and churches. Will you consider partnering with us to save lives?

If you have benefited from reading my book, I would greatly appreciate your reviews and recommendations on Facebook, Amazon, Kindle, Twitter and GoodReads.com, etc....AND if you have ideas on how we can better share the message of this book, please let us know. I'd also WELCOME your personal letters if you have found encouragement in this book.

To order additional books, inquire about bulk discounts, or to make a donation, please visit us at www.HopeDr.org and/or call 1-800-734-3439.

Stress and Grief Relief, Inc. is a 501(c)(3) non-profit organization (EIN: 95-4722033) committed to preventing suicide and its causes. Will you please join in this critical effort, become an instrument in God's hands and pray and help spread hope, save lives, and make a difference? With tremendous, heartfelt appreciation for your prayers and support, will you please now visit the website to make a tax deductible donation today: https://hopedr.org/donations/hopepartners/

As time permits, Dr. Joyce accepts speaking requests. If you would like to be notified when she may be in an area near you, please write to her or send an email with your name, location, and contact information.

Stress and Grief Relief, Inc.
355 West Mesquite Blvd. Suite C-70,
Mesquite, NV 89027
askwisdom@yahoo.com

Questions? Want more information?

Need a book? Know someone who really needs a book? Have a story to tell about how this book helped you or a loved one? Please write, call or email:

1-800-734-3439
askwisdom@yahoo.com
www.StressandGriefRelief.org or www.HopeDr.org

Please join us and become a Hope Partner and an instrument in God's hands, sharing *Amazing Heavenly Answers* with the world, as we work to help people thrive and survive with miraculous results. Please visit our Hope Partners page today: https://hopedr.org/donations/hopepartners/

Made in the USA
Las Vegas, NV
20 September 2023

77881210R00144